Understanding Men
and Health

This book should be returned by the last date stamped
above. You may renew the loan for a further period
if the book is not required by another reader.

Understanding Men and Health

Masculinities, Identity and Well-being

Steve Robertson

Open University Press

Open University Press
McGraw-Hill Education
McGraw-Hill House
Shoppenhangers Road
Maidenhead
Berkshire
England
SL6 2QL

email: enquiries@openup.co.uk
world wide web: www.openup.co.uk

and Two Penn Plaza, New York, NY 10121–2289, USA

First published 2007

A catalogue record of this book is available from the British Library

ISBN–13: 9780335221561 (pb) 9780335221578 (hb)
ISBN–10: 0335221564 (pb) 0335221572 (hb)

Library of Congress Cataloguing-in-Publication Data
CIP data applied for

Typeset by YHT Ltd, London
Printed in Poland EU by Pozkal
www.polskabook.pl

The **McGraw·Hill** Companies

I dedicate this book to my children, Raphael and Rachael, for the times when their smiles have helped me through and especially to my dad who continues to teach me so much about what it means to be a man.

'And on the masculine side of this whole wide world there's no 101% man.'
'101% Man', from the Album *Gaze* by 'The Beautiful South'.

Contents

Foreword

It is remarkable to see the rapid increase in interest in the health of men since the mid-1980s. We have moved from a position where there was almost complete silence on the subject, an absence that was reflected not only in policy and clinical practice but also within the academic community, to this now being recognized as an area of major importance.

The epidemiological data are compelling, with men showing higher levels of premature mortality in nearly all diseases that should affect men and women equally, more deaths as a result of suicide and risk taking and with an increased vulnerability to worsening social conditions, not just in the UK but on a global scale (White and Cash 2004; White and Holmes 2006).

These sex differences are important, epidemiological data do not explain why these inequalities exist or why the variations are so marked as a result of changes in social circumstances. To begin to answer these questions we need to shift our gaze. We must move away from making comparisons with women alone to a more detailed analysis of why men differ from each other, and to do this the focus moves from biological differences between males and females to the differences that are created through society's expectations of and cultural influences on men. When the lens turns towards men's gender we see a different picture; we have an obligation to start to investigate the notion of masculinity in its many guises (such that now we refer to its plural form 'masculinities' (Connell 1995)). We need to explore if 'being a man' influences our health choices and how the fluidity of the concept of masculinity affects health.

This can only be achieved through going out to men and listening to their stories as they share their experiences and expectations of health, their health practices and their relationship with the health care system. A caveat exists, though: this is not as simple as it seems! Which men should you speak to? How are you going to persuade them to talk to you? What questions are you going to ask? What sense are you going to make of what they have said? What theory underpins your conclusions? It takes a person like Steve, who is well steeped in the area, to be able to tackle such a challenge.

This authoritative text with its in-depth interviews with men from a number of diverse backgrounds provides invaluable insights into how men think about their health and health behaviour. This detailed analysis reinforces the need to recognize a dichotomy of men both being similar and different at the same time, with the charge that men don't care about their health being seen as problematic, but also realizing that not all men's health is managed in the same way.

This book needs to become essential reading for anyone working or studying in any health-related area for, if academics and practitioners do not understand what health means to men, then how can practice be truly informed? A further consideration is that Steve's work is located within a growing field of men's health that exists as a separate academic field in its own right. The scope of work that needs to be undertaken to come to understand fully the relationship men have with their own and others' health requires dedicated consideration within the academic and clinical domain.

Across the world we are seeing activity on men's health, from academic departments being developed to the success of organizations such as the Men's Health Forum in England and the European Men's Health Forum in raising the awareness of the public and politicians to the importance of targeting men's health specifically. Reinforced with the legal requirements of the Gender Equality Duty in the UK and the World Health Organization for Gender Mainstreaming, this whole area now sits within a broader debate on having equitable outcomes in health-care delivery.

The cost of the problems in men's health spreads wide, with implications across the whole of society. We have to look to a health service that is aware of its potential in supporting men to make better life choices and to provide services that can have a positive effect on their health and well-being and this text is a significant step on the way to addressing that goal.

Professor Alan White PhD RN

Acknowledgements

Many people have contributed to bringing this work into being. First and foremost thanks must go to the men and health professionals whose voices bring the book to life and who made time in their busy schedules to talk with me. Thanks also to the health service and local authority professionals who helped me establish links with those whose voices appear here. The original research was made possible through an NHS Executive Northwest Regional Fellowship Grant (RDO/33/54) and the book structure was envisaged and developed with support from an ESRC/MRC Interdisciplinary Postdoctoral Award (PTA–037–27–0021).

Professor Tony Gatrell and Dr Carol Thomas have provided both excellent academic guidance, detailed comment, and valued personal support at times when it was very much needed. Professor Bernie Carter has helped create the much-needed space for writing up this research into book form. Numerous colleagues at the Institute for Health Research, Lancaster University, and in the Department of Nursing, University of Central Lancashire have both inspired me and made me laugh through the research and writing process. Thanks also to my 'critical friends', Bob Williams, Brendan Gough and Ciara Kierans, for commenting on aspects of the book while in draft form, and to Professor Alan White for taking the time to read the work and write a foreword.

The author and the publishers would like to acknowledge the following:

- Lyrics quoted from *101% Man*. Words and music by Paul Heaton and David Rotheray, © Copyright 2003 Universal/Island Music Limited. Used by permission of Music Sales Limited. All Rights Reserved. International Copyright Secured.
- Use of material in Chapter 2 that was first published by Sage Publications Ltd: Robertson, S. (2006) Not living life in too much of an excess: lay men understanding health and well-being, *Health: An Interdisciplinary Journal for the Social Study of Health, Illness and Medicine* 10(2): 175–89, © Sage Publications Ltd.
- Use of material in Chapter 3 that was first published by Blackwell Publishing: Robertson, S. (2006) I've been like a coiled spring this last week: embodied masculinity and health. *Sociology of Health and Illness* 28(4): 433–56.

Introduction

When we think about 'men's health' what are the thoughts and images that come to mind? Do we think of athletes, exercise and six-packs? Is it corporate businessmen straining to combine success at work with a quality home life and collapsing at 50 with a heart attack? Do we simply think of male-specific illness or disease such as testicular and prostate cancer? Are we more likely to think of unhealthy behaviours, of alcohol and drug abuse, poor diet, fast driving and violence? Or do we think about mental well-being, of difficulties in emotional expression and associated suicide rates particularly for young men? Is it about men having to show themselves as strong, stoical and if so how does that account for the 'Man Flu' syndrome where (supposedly) a simple cold results in men taking rapidly to bed and needing to be tended to by a female partner?

'Men's Health' has become a popular and well-recognized term since the mid-1980s, yet it is obviously not a coherent and easily definable concept. Indeed, there is some discussion and debate concerning reaching an agreement about defining 'men's health' (White 2006). Nevertheless, a quick flick through newspapers, popular magazines, as well as health professional and academic literature, reveals a significant and increasing level of interest and concern in the area. A search on the Medline database using the term 'men's health', and limited to the years 1997 to 2007, returns over 370 papers. This compares to just over a hundred papers using the same term for the ten years prior to that – more than a threefold increase. These articles and academic books/papers often provide statistics that compare and contrast men's longevity with that of women's, or identify worrying trends in increases in male specific morbidity (such as testicular cancer, prostate disease, suicide rates) in order to highlight, either implicitly or explicitly, concerns about a 'crisis in men's health'. Yet such a 'crisis', if indeed one does exist, is not devoid of wider social context. Explanations for men's health in such works are often tied in to a wider debate on the influence of 'masculinity', its changing nature in late modernity that creates a 'crisis in masculinity', and the (usually negative) impact of these forces on men's health behaviours and outcomes. Men are variously presented as cavalier, uncaring and/or unconcerned about health matters and this is tied in to wider narratives of men as 'poor', or at best reluctant, users of health services, particularly health services designed to promote and maintain health. Yet they are also presented as 'redundant', 'lost', lacking direction and losing identity as the manufacturing industries diminish and more women move out of the domestic sphere and into paid employment in the new(er) service industries. This 'double whammy' constructs men simultaneously as 'irresponsible' in terms of health-related behaviours and as 'victims' of destructive processes of socialization that negatively impact on their health status; they are discursively situated as both 'risk takers' and those 'at risk'. This is highlighted well in the UK medical/ nursing literature where article titles such as 'Their own worst enemy' (Williamson 1995) and 'Men's health: unhealthy lifestyles and an unwillingness to seek help' (Griffiths 1996) contrast with others with titles such as 'Equal rights for men' (Fareed 1994), 'Men's health: don't blame the victims' (Essex 1996), and 'Inequality, discrimination and neglect: men's health' (Peate 2006).

Despite this surge in interest and concern about men's health, there remains, as Watson (2000: 2) has previously highlighted, a striking absence of knowledge relating to this that is 'grounded in the everyday experience of men themselves'. There are significant bodies of material and data that relate to: male medical conditions; epidemiology and sex differences in disease profiles; psychological measures of 'masculinity' and their relations to health behaviours; health policy and its impact on men's health behaviour and outcomes, and examples of health professional service development to address 'men's health' issues. Yet, in contrast to the growing, qualitative, empirical work on men's 'illness' experiences (for example Sabo and Gordon 1995; Cameron and Bernardes 1998; White 1999; Pateman and Johnson 2000; White and Johnson 2000; Chapple and Ziebland 2002; Riessman 2003; Gannon et al., 2004; Emslie et al. 2006) there is currently a minimal comparative body of qualitative empirical data relating to men's health experiences. Furthermore, there is increasing evidence to suggest that men's health experiences are also influenced by the thoughts and practices of those delivering (and indeed not delivering) particular health-related services as well as by men's own thoughts and behaviours (see, for example, Robertson 1998; Williams and Robertson 1999; Banks 2001; Seymour-Smith et al. 2002).

Purpose and format

This book is based upon the premise that health-related behaviours and experiences, or my preferred term, 'health practices', cannot be fully understood outside of the social context(s) within which they emerge. The overarching aim of the book is therefore to consider how the relationship between 'masculinities' and 'health practices' are shaped within, and by, particular social contexts. This is largely done through the critical exploration of lay men's and health professionals' own accounts. In taking this approach, this book adds further empirical information, grounded in men's own experiences, to the 'men's health' field. This book therefore aims to be of value to academics with an interest in gender, masculinities and health and of use to health practitioners in thinking about how to develop public health work further with men.

The way that I approached achieving this aim, the methodology and methods used and the people involved, provides the material for the rest of this introductory chapter. Chapter 1 considers in more detail the issues raised so far in this introduction. It locates the subject of men's health within the wider policy context and reviews the current literature and research on gender, masculinity and health. This is not an exhaustive research and policy review. Rather, it focuses predominantly on the situation within the UK but does draw on research and policy from other countries when appropriate. The latter part of Chapter 1 considers how the concept of 'masculinities' is to be understood, and how it will be used as a conceptualizing framework within the rest of the book. In particular, it introduces the concept of 'hegemonic masculinity' – a term that has gained wide appeal across various academic disciplines since the 1990s. The introduction and first chapter therefore provide contextualizing information for the empirical chapters that follow.

Chapter 2, begins to look specifically at the lay men and health professional accounts; the empirical data. It considers how the men, and to a lesser extent the health professionals, articulated ideas about what constituted health, how they understood and defined the concept, and how such abstract definitions become gendered in nature as they are transformed into actions, into social practices. It looks at the narratives around 'risk', 'responsibility', 'control' and 'release', key concepts in health promotion, and develops a framework for understanding the relationship between health and hegemonic masculinity. Embodiment has become a way of understanding bodies as more than just *objects*, 'physiological entities'. Rather, we are seen as 'embodied beings', where bodies are recognized as key sites of our *subjective* experience in everyday encounters and not simply as the physical vessel that our identity resides in.

Chapter 3 therefore uses the notion of embodiment, explicitly building on Watson's (2000) previous work (introduced in more detail in the following chapter), to explore how differing modes of male embodiment interact and how this interaction relates to men's health practices. In this way, the chapter theorizes from (rather than about) men's accounts of the body, and their bodily practices, and develops an argument that bodies need to be considered as both material (physical) and representational (symbolic, signifying and conveying shared emotions, information and feelings) if men's health practices are to be more adequately understood.

Chapter 4 considers the men's narratives around relationships and their impact on health. It draws on current literature and research on the sociology of the emotions, as well as limited research on gender, health and social capital, to make an argument that emotion for men is often communicated within and through action rather than being internally 'felt' or verbally articulated.

Chapter 5 expands the discussions initiated earlier (in Chapter 2) on responsibility for health and relates this directly to men's narratives on the role of health services. It explicitly covers discussions around the nature of health information and health screening services and how, when, where and why men do (or do not) engage with health-promoting services. It links the empirical data to discussions in the health promotion field about the rise of surveillance medicine.

The concluding chapter draws together the empirical and theoretical work presented and links this back to the current context of men's health. It recaps on the main points that emerge concerning the relationships between men, masculinity and health and in doing so develops suggestions for policy and practice and identifies potential areas for future research.

The key points made, and the relevance of the content for health practitioners, are presented at the end of each chapter.

Lay and professional narratives: methodology and method

The purpose of this section is to paint a broad brush-stroke picture (rather than providing the fine detail) of why and how the particular approach to collecting the accounts was adopted and executed in order to provide sufficient detail to allow a 'feel' for the project to develop without becoming too diverted from the subject content of the book.

Why lay narratives?

To some extent there could be said to be a 'so what' element to hearing about how people understand and experience 'health'. Taken simply, and at face value, whilst each individual can offer their particular thoughts or opinion, how can a small collection of such idiosyncratic views provide real and significant insight into a problem as complex and convoluted as the relationship between 'masculinities' and 'health'?

Blaxter (1997: 747) points out that lay talk about health and illness provides 'accounts of social identity'. In this way, people's talk about health is rarely, if ever, simply an objective description. Instead, such accounts convey, often unconsciously, what people wish to tell us about themselves. Take the following quote from one of the participants: 'If there is anything wrong with me I leave it to the body to repair itself. I'm not one if I get the sniffles, I don't take tablets, I don't take medicines. If I get the sniffles, I get the sniffles' (Hugh, CABS2).

Hugh is not *just* providing a straightforward description of his behaviour, he is telling something about himself, perhaps that he is virtuous in his use of health services, or that as a man he is strong, able to fight off simple colds without help from outside services. Clearly, it takes more than one short quote to understand the identity (or identities) that Hugh seeks to convey. Nevertheless, this demonstrates how identities are constructed and relayed through narratives about 'health'. In this sense, health is something that represents a range of practices as well as a state of being and also carries moral connotations (see also Cornwell 1984; Crawford 1984, 2006). As such, how it is conceptualized and accounted for, and indeed how, when and where various health practices are pursued or not, all provide insight into how various social identities are constructed and/or performed. Clearly, gender is one such aspect of social identity and previous research on gender and health has used lay men's and women's accounts to show how 'doing health' is a form of 'doing gender' (Saltonstall 1993). The 'doing' of gender, as West and Zimmerman (1987) explain, means understanding gender not as something that *we are* but as something that *we do*. We must continually socially reconstruct our gender in everyday encounters knowing that we are judged against society's standards of what are deemed appropriate feminine or masculine behaviours. The way that we 'do' health therefore also acts to construct and convey our gendered identity.

Yet, this 'social identity' is not merely a matter of individual identity; not merely a social psychology used to try to explain individual action. Rather, social identities are also collective, existing in places, spaces and historical moments. They are created and performed in interaction, within sets of social relationships, and thereby also become embedded in social structures. In this way, critical exploration of lay narratives can provide insight into questions of structure and agency; into the relationship between individuals and the wider social context within which they live. Popay and colleagues have begun to clarify the theoretical importance of lay knowledge in relation to public health research (Popay and Williams 1996), and health inequalities (Popay et al. 1998) and to develop empirical work that grounds this theoretical debate (Popay et al. 2003). Moreover, they have specifically shown how lay narratives about lived experiences can help illuminate 'the complex relationships between identity, agency and social structures' in relation to research into gender inequalities and health (Popay and Groves 2000: 85). In considering how best to move forward when researching gender inequalities in health, Annandale and Hunt (2000) also reinforce the need to incorporate more qualitative approaches that help understand people's health experiences within their social contexts rather than trying to reduce them to measurable aspects of people's knowledge and behaviour (see also Thomas 1999a).

The suggestion here is not that people's accounts of their lived experience are taken as incorrigible 'truths', accepted at face value as factual accounts.

Rather, they are also representational accounts that, in the process of their construction and telling, provide one perspective on how the identities people construct, and the actions they take, can shape, and also be shaped, both directly and indirectly, by powers invested within the social structures that surround them. This shaping may be conscious or subconscious but is nonetheless elucidated through the critical analysis of lay narratives.

Incorporating professional accounts

The issue of power within doctor–patient, lay–professional relationships has long been a topic of interest and study within the medical sociology field (see, for example, Turner 1987; Nettleton 1995). Much of this work has highlighted the dominance and precedence gained by medical/professional discourses over patient/lay accounts concerning health. However, research has also begun to suggest that this 'powerful professional'/'passive patient' dualism may be more complex than previously envisaged with acts of resistance to professional discourses and negotiated discourses being prevalent alongside 'submissive' patient encounters (see, for example, Lupton 1996, 1997; Ong and Hooper 2006). This is not to say that medical discourses do not continue to exert significant power and influence in late modernity, nor is it an attempt to downplay the material implications of such power differentials. Rather, it is to recognize how power that exists in a macro-social sense can become dispersed, or at least challenged, within micro-social encounters.

The lay–professional encounter is therefore a complex process that both relies on, and (re)constructs, aspects of social hierarchies, of social identities, and provides examples of how such hierarchies and identities are gendered in nature. Research by Seymour-Smith et al. (2002) suggests that men's health encounters within a primary care setting are influenced by how health professionals conceptualize issues around 'masculinity'. They show how professional actions can act to replicate and sustain, give primacy to and anticipate particular forms of masculine practices within the health-care setting.

In order to help understand more thoroughly the relationship between 'masculinity' and 'men's health practices', it therefore seems important to also explore professional narratives in order to consider how these two concepts might be coconstructed within the medical context. In short, it was felt to be important not only to understand how men conceptualized 'masculinity' and 'health' but also how health professionals think men conceptualize these and how professionals themselves construct this relationship.

Accessing and understanding narrative accounts

So far, we have considered the theoretical importance of lay and professional accounts in helping to elucidate the relationship between 'masculinity' and 'health practices' by their ability to link more adequately issues of structure and agency. Here we will look briefly at where and how narrative accounts were collected and interpreted. You will find short vignettes about each of the participants at the end of this introduction.

This project was geographically based in and around (within a 30 mile radius) the town of Blackpool in the north-west of England. Blackpool is historically popular as a seaside resort and continues to attract a significant number of tourists. The town centre is very much built around the leisure and tourism industry, consisting predominantly of hotels, bed-and-breakfast houses, amusement parks and arcades, as well as bars and nightclubs. It has a large gay community, both as residents and visitors, and a significant part of the leisure industry caters specifically for the 'gay scene'. The seasonal nature of the town can give the area an appearance of being somewhat bleak and run down in the winter months and also creates a significant transient population due to the seasonal nature of employment. Employment does vary, being mainly related to the tourism and leisure industry in the town centre and a mixture of small manufacturing and service-based employment in the sub-urbs. There is a great deal of wealth in some of the suburban and semi-rural towns and villages that surround Blackpool and therefore a great deal of contrast in the socio-economic circumstances of those living within and between these locations and the town centre. Consequently, there are wide variations in health outcomes across Blackpool and its suburbs. At 72.8 years, Blackpool has the second lowest average male life expectancy in England whereas surrounding localities (such as Wyre and Fylde) have rates higher than the national average (Office for National Statistics 2005a).

Within this community, covering a population of approximately 321,000 residents, the project intended to focus on men aged between 25–40 years. This age group is important for two main reasons in relation to men and health. First, it incorporates the age range of men who are amongst the lowest users of primary care (general practitioner) health services within England (Office for National Statistics 2002). This is often said to be representative of men's reluctance to care for their health and therefore postulated as one explanation for men's reduced longevity (see, for example, Courtenay 2000b; Banks 2001). Second, there are increasing concerns about specific issues with men of this age that impact on health and well-being. Two such major issues are suicide rates and obesity rates. Men in this age range are those with the highest rates of suicide within the UK (Office for National Statistics 2006a) and obesity rates are climbing amongst younger men and look set to continue to rise over the coming years (Zaninotto et al. 2006). The final selection of men included within the project had an age range of 27–43 years.

The phrase 'men's health' carries with it an almost inherent tendency to homogenize men. It encourages explanations that try to account for health (as outcome, as sets of beliefs, practices) amongst 'men' as a singular, distinct category. These explanations often rely on a notion of 'masculinity' that is to be understood as a set of shared characteristics, common to men, *as if* they are all the same. Yet, for those who work with men, or even if we stop and take time to think about men we know, it is clear that men's experiences and practices are rich and varied. The health experiences of gay men, men on low income, men with physical impairment and so forth are unlikely to be the same (Robertson 2000). 'Masculinity' coexists as a form of practice with other aspects of identity construction and management such as sexuality, ethnicity, disability, social class and so forth. With this in mind, I felt it important to look at lay accounts from a cross-section of men. The final group of men therefore consisted of seven gay men (one of whom was also disabled), six disabled men, and seven men self-identified as neither gay nor disabled. Other contextualizing information about the men is provided at the end of this chapter as vignettes. Names and other obviously identifying information have been altered but without losing the feel for the description of the person portrayed. The pseudonyms chosen are not meant to be signifiers of any sort.

Cornwell (1984) points out the difficulties involved in obtaining private rather than public accounts about health when conducting research. She suggests there is a need to complete more than one such interview in order to obtain more private accounts. The 20 men were therefore interviewed on two separate occasions with interviews lasting from 30 minutes to three hours (except for two gay men, originally interviewed together who were not available for the second interview).

In addition to these men, seven community health professionals, representing a range of disciplines, were interviewed. Brief contextualizing information about these professionals, again anonymized, is presented at the end of this chapter.

Once obtained, all interviews were fully transcribed and a process that looked for emerging themes within and across the interview narratives took place. Apart from one other emerging theme – that of sport and fitness – reported on elsewhere (Robertson 2003), the four empirical chapters of this book represent these emerging themes and their critical analysis.

A word on notation and quotation

The interview extracts used in this book are mainly quoted verbatim although interviewer interjections have sometimes been omitted. Where part of the verbatim text is omitted this is indicated by brackets and ellipses as follows [. . .]. Significant pauses or changes in conversation direction are shown by use of ellipses without brackets as follows ... Where points or words are emphasized this is shown by the use of *italics* and it is made clear at the end of the quote if this emphasis has been added rather than being emphasized by the participant. *Italics* are also used in the text as well as the quotes to emphasize points of key significance. Where conversations are presented the participants are shown by name and I am abbreviated to my initials, SR.

In addition to being identified by pseudonyms, the participants were also assigned a group code and a number (representing the order they were interviewed in within this group): health professionals were HP, gay men were GM, disabled men were DM and those men who did not identify specifically as gay or disabled were coded as CABS (Contingently Able-Bodied and Straight). This CABS notation is formulated as a means of recognizing that although the men currently do not identify as gay or disabled this is contingent on current circumstances and they may have previously, or may go on to identify, or be identified, as gay and/or disabled. As will become clear, these codes are not meant to suggest character types for these individuals but rather were used in recognition of the importance that people, including the participants themselves, attach to assigning themselves to particular identity groupings and how this may influence health practices. Neither are such groupings clearly bounded or mutually exclusive and, as the vignettes show, one man identified as both gay and disabled and two of the CABS had chronic illnesses but did not identify themselves as disabled men.

Participant vignettes

Lay men

Andrew – [GM7]. Thirty-seven-year-old gay man. After working in the caring professions when young, moved to Blackpool 15 years ago and has mainly been involved in bar work and management since then. Active in voluntary work for HIV/AIDS.

Bob – [CABS6]. Thirty-seven year old man. Moved around a lot with father's work as a boy, including spells abroad. Went into the army from school for several years and did numerous labouring and driving jobs since leaving the army. Has two children aged 11 and 8 and has recently divorced. Diagnosed with multiple sclerosis six years ago and has been in and out of work since then, including a period of retraining to work with computers. Enjoys outdoor pursuits and active hobbies.

David – [GM1]. Twenty-eight-year-old gay man. Moved to Blackpool several years ago. In the 18 months between the first and second interview David went from being self-employed to managing a leisure venue. Also in this period he moved in with a partner and, following the breakdown of this relationship, became a lodger in a house with gay friends he has known for some time. Does voluntary work around gay and lesbian safety issues and HIV/AIDS.

Daniel – [CABS7]. Thirty-five-year-old graduate, currently working in the public sector in child care services and has commenced a part-time course to gain a formal vocational qualification in this area of work. Father died when he was seven years old, grew-up in a large city in the north-west of England and at 18 moved to Blackpool and then around the north of England working in sales, outdoor pursuits, studying, before settling back in Blackpool. Broke up from a six-year, cohabiting relationship recently and had a tentative relationship with new female partner by the time of the second interview. Enjoys active outdoor activities and sports.

Edward – [GM2]. Forty-two-year-old single, gay man. Moved to Blackpool 14 years ago seeking work. Worked mainly in hotel bar and management until being diagnosed HIV positive, now not formally employed but does some consultancy work. Previously very active in voluntary HIV/AIDS charity work although less so in recent years.

Francis – [CABS1]. A twenty-nine-year-old, works in the civil service and has done since leaving school. Francis was engaged at the time of the first interview and had moved from his parents' house to live with his fiancée by the time of the second interview. Has a daughter from a previous relationship but did not discuss level of contact with her.

Frank – [DM6]. Thirty-three-year-old disabled man, grew-up in Blackpool but recently moved 30 miles away. Has an hereditary muscle-wasting disease, becoming gradually more impaired, uses a wheelchair outdoors and has some difficulties with balance and limb strength. Married with three children from present relationship and four from two previous relationships. Not formally employed as studying at time of first interview but had put this on hold by the time of the second interview due to the demands of the youngest child (only two weeks old at time of first interview). Younger brother of Quinn (see below).

Gary – [GM3]. Forty-three-year-old gay man who has lived in Blackpool all his life. Currently lives with partner whom he has been with for 18 months. He works as a skilled labourer since serving an apprenticeship on leaving school. He was diagnosed as HIV positive five years ago. Describes himself as healthy, and enjoys exercising at the gym.

Hugh – [CABS2]. Thirty-three-year-old. Grew up in a run-down town in the north-west of England and went into the army from school where he spent 11 years and trained as a chef. Has lived in Blackpool for five years. He continues to work as a chef and is married with two young children.

Kiaran – [GM4]. Thirty-eight-year-old gay man. Has worked in the public sector caring professions, mainly with the elderly, since leaving school and also does voluntary work around gay and lesbian mental health and well-being. He has lived in Blackpool for the last four years, was previously in a heterosexual marriage, is now living with Neil and they have been together two years.

Larry – [CABS4]. Thirty-year-old man. Works in telecommunication sales and went from being employed to self-employed between the first and second interviews. During the research Larry became separated from his wife who then moved a significant distance away with their 2-year-old son and Larry found this situation very difficult. He was diagnosed as an insulin-dependent diabetic in his early 20s.

Martin – [CABS3]. Twenty-seven year old, who returned to the family home in Blackpool suburbs after graduating in science a few years ago. Works as an account manager in a small local business but hopes to move to London with his girlfriend in the near future. Father died of skin cancer when Martin was very young. Enjoys participating on a regular basis in a variety of sports and exercise.

Neil – [GM5]. Thirty-year-old gay man. Works in a bed and breakfast, lives with his partner, Kiaran, and hopes to return to college shortly. Moved to Blackpool six years ago with work.

Owen – [CABS6]. Thirty-years old. Born and raised in a Blackpool suburb and has been an office worker since leaving school. Took voluntary redundancy during the course of the research and is hoping to gain entry into the health professions. Involved in voluntary health work. Married for three years with a 1-year-old daughter.

Peter – [DM1]. Twenty-nine-year-old disabled man. Involved in an accident ten years ago that has left him paralysed from the mid-chest. Worked in the public sector for local government at the first interview but this contract ended and he had just begun a new position as a training coordinator for a private company specializing in caring services by the time of the second interview. Peter is married with young twins. Very active in disability sports.

Quinn – [DM2]. Thirty-six-year-old disabled man. Born and raised in Blackpool but spent some time in care as a teenager. Has hereditary muscle-wasting disease and is now almost permanently in a wheelchair and is also beginning to lose upper body strength. Has only been employed for very short periods. Active in wheelchair basketball and enjoys long-distance sponsored wheelchair pushes. Married, no children.

Ron – [DM3]. Thirty-four-year-old disabled man. Following accident in his early 20s he developed an extreme clotting disorder resulting in numerous thrombosis and mini-strokes. The amount of impairment varies with Ron being relatively active some days but unable to leave the house on others. Married since before the accident he has two teenage children. He worked in the brewery trade, but now does part-time office work as a civil servant.

Tony – [DM5]. Thirty-two-year-old man describes himself as disabled and gay. He has an impairment that makes speech and mobility difficult. He walks around his own home but uses a wheelchair if going out any distance and employs between seven and eight carers to help meet his physical needs. He is self-employed and describes himself as having a 'very active social life' although this depends on appropriate carers being able to take him out.

Vernon – [DM4]. Forty-three-year-old disabled man. Originally from a large north-west city, he has lived in Blackpool for over 18 years. He had a leg amputated through cancer ten years ago and is gradually losing the use of his other leg due to severe disc problems in his back and associated loss of sensation in this leg. Now he is an almost permanent wheelchair user. Currently he is not working; previously he was a skilled labourer. He is active in several disability sports. Married for 20 years; no children.

Wayne – [GM6]. Thirty-nine-year-old gay man. Has lived in Blackpool for 16 years. Works in horticulture and this sometimes entails periods away from Blackpool. He is the partner of Andrew whom he has been with for two years, although they have known each other much longer. Involved in local HIV/AIDS charity work.

Health professionals

Adam – [HP1]. Male district nurse, late 40s. Has run well-man and vasectomy clinics in the past.

Collette – [HP2]. Female health visitor, mid-50s. Says she has little professional involvement with male clients except occasional contact with fathers around issues such as parenting skills, post-natal depression (in female partners) and child protection.

Dawn – [HP5]. Female practice nurse, mid-40s. Sees male clients usually in the context of vaccination or diabetic clinics and new patient checks (a health check carried out when a patient first registers with a GP practice).

Eve – [HP6]. Female practice nurse, late 40s. Main involvement with men as clients is in a diabetic clinic and new patient checks.

Fiona – [HP7]. Female GP, mid-30s. Predominantly involved with men when acutely unwell and attending general surgery because of this.

Ian – [HP4]. Male community psychiatric nurse, early 40s. Sees men mainly when they have been referred, often for alcohol misuse and/or depression.

He says relationship issues constitute a significant part of his workload with men.

John – [HP3]. Male GP, early 40s. Tends to see men as clients only for episodes of acute illness.

1 The current context of men's health and the role of masculinities

Introduction

So far we have considered briefly the importance of undertaking this project, how it was approached, and have learned a little about the people involved. However, before considering what the men and health professionals had to say, we need first to put this in context. The critical analysis of the lay men's and health professionals' accounts provided in the chapters that follow involves examining these narratives in the light of previous and current policy and research on men's health in the UK. The first section of this chapter therefore concentrates on the historical and current policy context, highlighting why there is a concern about men's health, what has been done, or not, to address it and where the problems might lie with current approaches. The second section looks at what research has been completed in relation to men and their health and describes briefly work within the social sciences that has taken a variety of approaches to exploring men's health practices and outcomes.

As this book intends specifically to explore this relationship of 'masculinity' to health practices it is also important to show how 'masculinity/ masculinities' were understood within the project and used as a framework for the critical analysis of the narrative accounts provided. The third section of this chapter therefore examines how masculinity/masculinities have been conceptualized within previous literature and research and considers the implications of such conceptualizations in relation to health.

Defining the men's health field

Concern about 'men's health', which can act as a stimulus for influencing policy and its implementation, stems from a variety of epidemiological data. While not wishing to replicate all of this data here, it is important to point out some of the main concerns that are frequently raised in the current literature and discussions on men's health. These concerns are threefold relating to male mortality, morbidity, and health-related behaviours and are summarized below:

Box 1.1 Mortality, morbidity and 'behaviour'

- Average life expectancy for men in the UK is approximately four years less than it is for women (Office for National Statistics 2006b).
- Many of these 'lost years' for men, in the UK and across Europe, can be accounted for by the comparatively higher rates of death in younger men (White and Banks 2004).
- The causes of male death vary greatly with age. Accidents, injury and poisoning, along with suicide, account for almost 60 per cent of deaths in men between 15–34 years whereas heart disease and cancers are the greatest cause of death for men aged 35–54 years in the UK (Lloyd 2001).
- Significant inequalities in life expectancy between men exist in relation to social class and geographical location (White and Cash 2003; White et al. 2005).
- Men have a higher proportion of deaths than women across a wide range of major disease classification groups (White and Cash 2003) and are twice as likely as women both to develop and die from the ten most common cancers affecting both sexes (Men's Health Forum 2004a).
- Rates of testicular cancer have more than doubled in the UK between 1979 and 2002 (Office for National Statistics 2005b).
- The number of diagnosed cases of prostate cancer has significantly increased since the mid-1980s (although mortality rates have remained fairly constant) and it accounts for 23 per cent of all new male cancer diagnoses (Cancer Research UK 2006).
- Suicide amongst men in the UK has significantly increased in the 25–44 year age group in the last 30 years. Although no longer rising, it has remained consistently high amongst this age group for the last ten years (Office for National Statistics 2006b).
- Men in the UK are significantly more likely to be overweight/obese than women (Office for National Statistics 2003).
- Men in the UK are less likely than women to consume the recommended five daily portions of fruit and vegetables and more likely to have a higher than recommended salt intake (Office for National Statistics 2006b).
- Men in the UK are more likely than women to drink above recommended amounts, to binge drink, and to take illicit drugs (Office for National Statistics 2006b).
- Whilst overall rates of smoking continue to decline, prevalence remains higher amongst men than women in the UK (Office for National Statistics 2006b).
- In the UK, young men aged 16–24 years are the greatest victims of violent crime with 12.6 per cent having been assaulted in the last year (Home Office 2006).
- In the UK in 2004, men outnumbered women as offenders across all crime categories by more than four to one (Home Office 2005).

Comparative statistics from other developed countries show similar patterns and therefore suggest similar concerns. It is important to note that these statistics are not the only causes of concern raised in relation to men and their health and comprehensive work in the US shows that 'males of all ages are more likely than females to engage in over 30 behaviours that increase the risk of disease, injury, and death' (Courtenay 2000: 81). Clearly, such factors interrelate. For example, alcohol and smoking rates are also linked to social class and thereby to inequalities in mortality rates from alcohol and smoking related deaths not only between the sexes but also between men from different income groups.

Already, we can see there is some debate concerning what comes under the umbrella of 'men's health'. In a review of men's health literature in the UK, Lloyd (1996) suggests three prominent definitions: That men's health is:

- *biological* – about male specific anatomy and physiology;
- *risk-taking* – about men's engagement in potentially dangerous behaviours; and
- related to *masculinity* – the processes of being or becoming a man usually negatively influence men's health practices and outcomes.

It is increasingly common to find recognition that health practices and outcomes for men result from a combination of factors (for recent examples see Doyal 2000, 2001; Peate 2004; White 2006) and definitions of men's health have tried to capture these. In Australia, for instance, US definitions of women's health were drawn upon and adopted by certain groups to suggest that: 'a men's health issue is a disease or condition unique to men, more prevalent in men, more serious among men, for which risk factors are different for men or for which different interventions are required for men' (Fletcher 2001: 68).

However, the Men's Health Forum in England has highlighted how this definition fails to consider the wider social and political determinants of health. In response, and to also ensure the inclusion of boys as well as men, they define a *male* health issue as:

> ... one arising from physiological, social, cultural or environmental factors that have a specific impact on boys or men and/or where particular interventions are required for boys or men in order to achieve improvements in health and well-being at the individual or population level.
>
> (Men's Health Forum 2004a: 5)

This definition is more embracing, allowing scope for thinking about men's health issues as more than something that relates to individual or even groups of men. For example, it allows us to view domestic violence as a men's health issue as it requires particular interventions (for both men and women) to improve the health and well-being of men and women as both perpetrators or survivors of such violence. What seems to be the case, as Sabo (2000: 133) highlights, is that a theoretical distinction can be drawn between *men's health* and *men's health studies*. The former has an often uncritical (but nonetheless important) focus on 'organismic functions, physical vitality or susceptibility to illness' whereas the latter refers to 'the systematic analysis of men's health and illness that takes gender and gender health equity into theoretical account.' In short, it allows us to understand and explore male health issues in the context of gendered relations, a point we shall return to in the third section of this chapter and one that is key to the arguments made in this book. For now, we shall concentrate on how these concerns about men's health and health practices are reflected and implemented, or not, within UK policy.

The current policy context of men's health

Whilst initiatives that aim to improve men's health in the UK have a history dating back to the early 1980s, these activities initially tended to be localized and ad hoc (see Robertson 1995). It is generally recognized that the main policy driver for highlighting and addressing male health concerns at a national level followed the publication of the 1992 annual report of the Chief Medical Officer. As Luck et al. (2000) point out, the inclusion in this report of a specific chapter on the 'health of men' was the first official recognition that men's health should be on the UK political agenda and therefore an issue of national concern.

In theory, this report laid the groundwork for taking a more coherent and co-ordinated response to addressing the health of men in the UK with regions being urged to 'investigate ways to improve the health of men over the next few years' (Department of Health 1993). However, in practice, regional and local responses to this call for action varied. Luck et al. (2000: Chapter 8) provide a detailed study of the innovations that were forthcoming from some parts of the health service at a regional and local level in the period following this report. More common though was a non-response from health services to this call and a national survey of Directors of Public Health and Chief Administrative Medical Officers at this time showed that they ranked men's health twelfth out of a possible 13 suggested priority groups (MORI 1995).

The reasons why this national call was not directed into clear national policy directives/strategies, or even into greater action at regional and local levels, are undoubtedly complex. Certainly the way the government encouraged local health promotion activity, through the *Health of the Nation* framework (Department of Health 1992) and 1990 GP contract (Department of Health 1989), meant that a great number of primary care services began to offer 'well-man' clinics during the 1990s as they were recompensed for delivering such services. However, little, if any, consideration was given as to how effective such services might be in terms of the number of men attracted, whether they reached those men with the greatest health needs, or whether these needs could be met through such an approach. Reviews of well-man clinics suggest that they are not generally successful in attracting men (White 2001) and when they do it tends to be men from higher socio-economic groups, even when specifically set up in areas of deprivation (Brown and Lunt 1992). Others have also suggested that such clinics, and the 'health checks' they offer, are limited in their ability to address the wider psychological and social issues that constitute the totality of men's health (Robertson 1995; Piper 1997; Williams and Robertson 2006).

The change of government in the UK in 1997 created opportunities to develop and take men's health policy and practice in new directions. The publication of The Acheson Report (Acheson 1998), *Saving Lives: Our Healthier Nation* (Department of Health 1999) and *Tackling Health Inequalities* (Department of Health 2003) signified a shift (at least rhetorically) in government direction, moving away from individual, health-promotion approaches, and towards public health models that bring issues around inequalities in health, including gender inequalities in health, centre stage. Within this inequalities agenda, the Department of Health has shown some specific concern with, and commitment to, addressing men's health. Speeches made by ministers for public health (Department of Health 2000, 2004), the inclusion of men's health projects in the Health Development Agency's (HDA) annual business plans, and the formation of an All Party Parliamentary Group on Men's Health, all suggest government recognition that men's health is part of the inequality agenda.

However, the Men's Health Forum (MHF), the biggest independent UK body that works for the development of health services that meet men's needs, has consistently raised concerns about the level of Department of Health commitment to actively and coherently implement this policy rhetoric. Their document, *Getting it Sorted*, sets out a policy programme for men's health (Men's Health Forum 2004a) and highlights how several national strategic health initiatives – such as the NHS Cancer Plan and the various National Service Frameworks – often fail to take gender sufficiently into account. This, they say, suggests 'that men's health issues are not taken as seriously as they should be by the Department of Health' (p. 8). The current UK policy approach to ensuring that services more consistently recognize and act sensitively to gender issues is to use a 'gender mainstreaming' model. Based on World Health Organization (WHO) recommendations, this process: '... promotes the integration of gender concerns into the formulation, monitoring and analysis of policies, programmes and projects, with the objective that women and men achieve the highest health status' (World Health Organization 2001).

In the UK, the opportunity to develop this approach is going to be further assisted by the implementation of a 'Gender Duty'. This duty became law in 2007 and requires all public authorities, including councils and health services, to eliminate discrimination and promote equality of opportunity between men and women. It remains to be seen how this will be implemented and the effect it will have for promoting gender sensitive health services for men as well as women.

It cannot be denied that, at a local level, there has been a significant increase in the amount and type of health work aimed at engaging men in the UK since the mid-1990s. Media interest and concern, generated through the determination and drive of organizations like the Men's Health Forum (MHF) and their establishment of events such as men's health week, have played a large part in this increased activity. In recognition of the historical difficulties experienced in getting men to attend health checks at GP surgeries, a raft of innovative approaches have been developed to take health services out to where men already gather and examples of these are provided on the 'projects database' at the MHF Web site (see also Davidson and Lloyd 2001). Yet, much of this local men's health activity remains vulnerable when funding is not specifically ring-fenced or is time limited and 'hard outcome' dependent. Despite clear health needs, it is often difficult for practitioners to argue their case for sustainable service delivery for men's health initiatives when government commitment remains ambiguous and ill-defined and short-term targets take preference over cultural change and community development approaches.

Two papers (Robertson and Williamson 2005; Williams and Robertson 2006) make suggestions as to why, despite this development of innovative approaches to reach men 'where they are at', current services still do not seem to impact on the statistics provided at the outset of this chapter. Three main reasons are identified in these papers. First, much of this 'new' activity uses aspects of 'masculinity' to engage with men and it is suggested that this runs the risk of inadvertently legitimizing and thereby replicating some potentially destructive aspects of men's behaviour (see also Robertson 2003). Second, they suggest that much of the practical engagement of health professionals with men, the focus of face-to-face encounters, continues to be based on the physical body and lifestyle change. Yet, this does not necessarily match men's own concerns (see also Watson 2000) and does little to 'ensure that men have the skills to cope with failing relationships or to avoid resorting to violence when faced with situations of conflict in private or public' (Williams and Robertson 2006: 27) – both considerable public health issues. Finally, there is recognition that we still have a limited evidence base in relation to men and health, particularly in relation to men's preventative health practices. Not only is the research base limited but there has been little coherent collation of the evidence that is available and the implications of this for practice. It is to consideration of this available evidence that we now turn.

What do we know about men and health?

Before addressing this question, it is necessary to first consider what is not being discussed here. It is often difficult to make a distinction between health and ill health, but this section will not be looking at the latter. The opening of this chapter has already provided some 'headline data' in terms of male mortality, morbidity and health practices and further epidemiological information is readily available from official statistics sources and existing men's health reports and texts (for example White and Cash 2003; Kirby et al. 2004; White 2006). Recent years have seen a significant increase in qualitative studies that explore men's ill-health experiences and how masculinity facilitates and inhibits specific behaviours and practices in these ill-health contexts. These contexts include coronary heart disease (Helgeson 1995: White 1999; White and Johnson 2000), prostate diseases (Cameron and Bernardes 1998; Chapple and Ziebland 2002; Gray 2003; Gannon et al. 2004), testicular cancer (Gordon 1995; Mason and Strauss 2004), multiple sclerosis (Riessman 2003), depression (Brownhill et al. 2005; Emslie et al. 2006), coeliac disease (Hallert et al. 2003) and fibromyalgia (Paulson et al. 2002). Together, this research supports Charmaz's (1995: 286) claim that: 'A man can gain a strengthened or a diminished identity through experiencing illness. These are not mutually exclusive categories. Men often move back and forth depending on their situations and their perceptions of them.'

However, there is significantly less research and evidence looking at men's *health* experiences and practices in the context of their everyday life. It is this body of literature that I wish to consider here. This work can be split into two main 'types': psychological approaches that measure aspects of 'masculinity' and relate these to health outcomes/practices; and sociological approaches that attempt to explore how men understand 'health' and the relationship of this to varied social contexts. We shall consider each of these in turn.

Masculinity scales and role theory

Psychologists trying to understand the relationship of men to their health have often attempted to 'operationalize' the concept of 'masculinity' as a variable in order to ascertain its relationship to health outcomes or health-related practices. This has been done predominantly through the use of psychological scales, perhaps the best known being Bem's Sex Role Inventory (BSRI) (Bem 1974, 1981). The BSRI asks people to assess how true 60 personality characteristics (predetermined as being 'masculine' or 'feminine') are for them on a seven-point scale. An assessment is then made and people characterized as: 'high masculine/low feminine', 'low masculine/high feminine', 'high masculine/high feminine' (androgynous) and 'low masculine/low feminine' (undifferentiated). In the UK, Annandale and Hunt (1990) used the BSRI and correlated it with physical measures of health (height, blood pressure and self-assessment), indicators of mental health (using a recognized psychological scale and self-assessment), self-assessed general health and health service utilization (number of GP visits in the last year). The results challenged the common-sense notion of 'masculinity' being detrimental to health with those who scored as 'highly masculine' (these could be men or women) having better self-reported measures of mental and physical health and lower rates of health service utilization.

Pleck (1995) has also reviewed research using scales that measure how much a man has internalized, or holds to, traditional notions of masculinity; that is what Pleck terms gender ideology as opposed to the gender orientation of the BSRI. Whilst these masculinity scales vary, they have been used to link masculinity with the following: lower levels of social support; less help seeking for psychological problems; lower levels of same-sex intimacy and higher rates of homophobia; increased alcohol and drug use; less consistent use of condoms; increased cardiovascular stressors; more sexual partners; and a belief that relationships between men and women are inherently adversarial.

There is, then, conflicting evidence from these scales about whether 'masculinity' confers advantages or disadvantages in terms of health practices and outcomes. This is possibly because of the different ways that 'masculinity' is conceptualized and operationalized in these studies. The journal *Psychology of Men and Masculinity* fills every edition with empirical papers showing how various versions of masculinity/gender scales relate to a range of social indicators, many of which have public health implications.

Such scales rely heavily, theoretically, on 'role theory' and differentiating sex-roles in order to formulate the (usually Likert) scales then used to measure 'masculinity' or its characteristics. As we shall see in the third section of this chapter, this way of conceptualizing or operationalizing gender and masculinity has been heavily criticized, particularly by sociologists. It is to sociological studies that we now turn.

Sociological studies and the voices of lay men

There is a significant amount of quantitative research, based on large-scale data sets, that has examined health differentials for men and women in relation to social structures (for example Arber 1997; Dunnell et al. 1999), to social relationships (Fuhrer et al. 1999), to social roles (Arber 1991), to work (Emslie et al. 1999) and to income (Rahkonen et al. 2000) to name but a few. These studies are increasingly showing more similarities than differences in physical morbidity amongst men and women, certainly until the age of 70 years.

Other survey work from within the UK complements the above data by directly asking lay men (and women) about their ideas and practices relating to health. The Health and Lifestyles Survey (HALS) (Blaxter 1990; Cox et al. 1997) suggests that men in the age band represented in this book most commonly thought of 'health' as a normal, ordinary state and associated it very much with athleticism and fitness (Blaxter 1990: 20, 24). Very few men in these studies defined health in terms of social relationships, communication with others or as 'psycho-social well being' but regularly related it to being able to function, particularly in paid work (Blaxter 1990: 26–8).

An ESRC-funded survey (Sharpe and Arnold 1999), involving men aged 25–35 years, showed that the majority of men denied that work was more important than their health yet would not take time off, confide in their boss or look for another job if they felt work was affecting their health. Peer pressure seemed important in encouraging health practices such as smoking and alcohol consumption and in dissuading men from making healthy dietary choices. Discussions about weight and fitness levels seemed acceptable, but talking directly about health or illness was seen as 'wussy' and was thought to indicate signs of weakness. Perhaps because of this, the research suggests that men distance themselves from health issues and their own health needs. Many of the men also felt overwhelmed by health information that often seemed contradictory, and they had concerns about how health information was transmitted.

Survey work with young people aged 15–17 years (Brannan et al. 1994) produced some interesting results that might conflict with stereotypical assumptions about young men. When asked to rank the top three from a series of items that were 'the most important things in life' a higher proportion of young men than young women ranked health in the top three (it being second for the young men and fourth for the young women on aggregate – Brannan et al. 1994: 71) although the young women were more likely to worry about their health. This work also incorporated the views of a number of parents and it is interesting to note that parents were more likely to report young men's health as being good compared to that of young women. With regard to specific health practices, alcohol consumption and drug taking were very similar among the young men and women. However, the young men engaged in a significantly higher amount of physical activity and were less likely to smoke (17 per cent compared with 30 per cent of young women). The men in the study, both fathers and the young men themselves, were more likely to view health as being within their individual control and young men were more likely to self-report good health.

Drawing on data from the west of Scotland Twenty–07 study, researchers from the MRC Social and Public Health Sciences Unit at Glasgow University have completed several surveys to consider sex differences in morbidity and GP consultation rates. Work by Macintyre et al. (1996) made comparisons between the reporting of a range of symptoms and identified diseases. For the majority of symptoms and diseases there was no statistically significant difference in reporting rates between men and women. Where there were statistically significant differences it was not always women who reported higher rates. For example, whereas women reported higher rates of 'malaise' symptoms and arthritis, men reported more 'trouble with eyes' and digestive disorders. The overall conclusion was that gender differences in morbidity and its reporting are complex and dependent on the particular symptoms and conditions being experienced. This work was expanded by Macintyre et al. (1999) through the collection of data regarding their response to a standard question on long-standing illness. Overall, no statistically significant sex differences were found in the reporting of conditions or their severity. This research was further supported by work undertaken by Hunt et al. (1999). Here, data were collected regarding GP consultation rates and the self-reporting of chronic illness and severity of symptoms in the previous year. The reporting of chronic illness followed the pattern of Macintyre et al. (1996) research, with women reporting more musculoskeletal and mental health problems and men reporting more digestive and cardiovascular problems. However, for all condition types, except mental health problems, similar levels of symptom severity did not produce any significantly different level of GP consultation, again challenging the view that 'women are simply more likely to consult a GP than men irrespective of underlying morbidity' (Macintyre et al. 1996: 96). A recent review of the literature on men and help-seeking raises further questions about suggested simplistic relationships between sex differences in help-seeking (Galdas et al. 2005).

Such survey work of the kinds described above can be limited in helping us understand more about the aggregate data obtained. In recognition of this, a further genre of qualitative sociological work obtaining in-depth lay accounts about health has developed. Several of the key early studies into lay accounts of health focused exclusively on women's lay perspectives (Pill and Stott 1982; Blaxter and Paterson 1982; Currer 1986; Calnan 1987). Two notable exceptions to this were the work carried out by Crawford (1984) in the US and that carried out by Cornwell (1984) in the UK both of which included men and women. Crawford's work was both original and vital in highlighting the moral character of lay perspectives, yet it failed to give due consideration to the gendered nature of such accounts. Cornwell's work also highlighted the moral nature of lay accounts of health and illness but drew out some gendered differences in how such accounts affected everyday life. For example, she explored how men could legitimately be 'off work' when unwell whereas women, as keepers of the home and family health, were (morally) required to continue their labour under similar circumstances.

Qualitative studies that exclusively focus on male lay perceptions of health remain relatively few in number. Mullen's (1993) work on Glaswegian men and health was possibly one of the earliest to provide information specifically on male lay perspectives of health. His findings about how men understood 'health' echoed many of those outlined in the HALS surveys discussed above. However, he had additional findings relating to: the emphasis that the men placed on the effect of the environment on health, the emphasis the men placed on the relationship between activity and health, and the fact that physical appearance as an indicator of health *was* of concern to the men in the study. In particular, his work concentrated on men's tobacco and alcohol use and highlighted how these were used as a release from stress, allowing men to continue to function, this functioning being seen in turn as a positive measure of health. It is also notable in Mullen's work that family life, particularly that with children, provided the men with alternatives to drinking and smoking and 'drew' them 'towards responsible conviviality' (Mullen 1993: 177).

This raises questions about how men understand 'health' differently as an abstract concept, when they rarely, if ever, discuss it in terms of social relationships (Blaxter 1990: 26–8, Mullen 1993: 60), and how they explore or explain specific health practices through their lived experiences. Saltonstall (1993), in the US, has explored this notion of differences between abstract concepts of 'health' and concrete health practices. One of the most notable findings is that although the male and female participants had similar views regarding what constituted health (as an abstract concept), these views 'dissipated into gender specific forms when translated into action in the everyday world' (Saltonstall 1993: 9). Specifically, men were more concerned with the functionality of the body (body-as-subject) as an indication of health whereas women were more concerned with the body's appearance (body-as-object) as an indicator of good health. Similarly, in relation to health practices, although the participants shared ideas about what was required in order to maintain health, their actions in the everyday world 'were guided and constrained by social norms and situations' (Saltonstall 1993: 11); that is, what was seen as appropriate for an individual as male or female. In conclusion, Saltonstall (1993: 12) suggests that 'The doing of health is a form of doing gender'.

Watson (1993) has carried out similar work to that of Saltonstall within the UK. His research is based on sequential interviews with 30 men and observation of the 'cultural event' of a well-man clinic. He focuses on health as an embodied concept in that the practices that men engage in – whether it be work, 'pumping iron' down the gym, or over-eating and sustained heavy drinking – are made visible, inscribed, on the physical body. When discussing issues of control and health, the men in the study felt that the body 'put itself in order', it alerted the men to excesses and there was a general 'if it works, don't fix it' approach to body maintenance (Watson 1993: 249). Health practices, particularly exercise, were often seen as being used merely to give the appearance of health for self-image rather than being for the creation or sustaining of health directly. In further exploring the same empirical data, Watson (2000) suggests that, through the interviews and observation, different forms of embodiment can be distinguished, allowing the development of a 'male body schema' in the context of health (see Table1.1).

Table 1.1   Watson's (2000) 'male body schema'

Normative embodiment	'Normal', 'standard' or idealized accounts of bodily shape(s).
Pragmatic embodiment	The functional use of a 'normal everyday body' in order to fulfil specific roles ('father', 'husband', 'worker') required in the social world.
Experiential embodiment	The point of contact of social and physical boundaries, the primary site for experience of emotion and physicality.
Visceral embodiment	The indirect biological processes, usually unconsciously experienced, that support bodily function and, to an extent, determine bodily shape.

He highlighted how, whereas health professionals often focused on visceral embodiment (accessed via experiential and normative embodiment), men themselves were more focused on pragmatic embodiment, on maintaining a functioning body in everyday life that allowed them to fulfil gender specific roles and expectations. It is this discrepancy in focus that Watson claims is responsible, at least in part, for the lack of success of health promotion work with men. We shall return to Watson's work, particularly the 'male body schema', in some detail in Chapter 3.

Research on gender, masculinity, social capital and health (Sixsmith and Boneham 2001; Sixsmith et al. 2001) suggests that health, for men, is a particularly private affair, not something 'done' in the public arena, with health talk being perceived as 'feminine' and therefore at odds with masculine identity. This work also explores how age, place and space affects concerns with masculine identity, social relations and thereby health. In this sense 'masculine' identity and its impact on health and well-being needs to be understood as being fluid, changing over time, and complex, dependant on other aspects of identity and wider social structures.

This suggestion of complexity and fluidity is further recognized in recent research emerging from Scotland. O'Brien et al. (2005) completed a study, based on focus group interviews with diverse groups of men, which explored the context of men's help-seeking for health concerns. A rhetorical reluctance to seek help was part of a collective representation of masculine identity, especially amongst the younger men, but one could actively depart from this rhetorical reluctance to engage with health services through a 'negotiated reasoning for this departure' (O'Brien et al. 2005: 514). What O'Brien et al. (2005) suggest is that men need a means of legitimating engagement with health services and that this can be done through the need to preserve or restore other aspects of masculinity (for example to fulfil gendered social roles, maintain sexual performance and so forth). They further suggest therefore that choosing, or not, to seek help for health concerns depends on negotiating a 'hierarchy of threats to masculinity' (O'Brien et al. 2005: 514). Likewise, amongst a group of older Scottish men, McVittie and Willock (2006: 788) also found that delay in seeking help 'can be viewed as reflecting tran-sitions in identity rather than hegemonic masculinity itself'. They suggest that the men did not simply move from a hegemonic identity to a 'sub-ordinated' masculine identity when faced with symptoms of ill health, but tended to oscillate between these using a 'time will tell' discourse to maintain a state of transitional identity. This obviously becomes increasingly difficult as bodily fragmentation makes it more difficult to sustain a hegemonic masculine identity. As we shall see throughout this book, such negotiations as described in these two studies are not limited to processes of seeking help (or not) but are also present in other contexts to support adherence, or not, to healthy and health promoting practices.

Masculinity/masculinities and health

So far we have considered the policy context and looked at some of the available research evidence concerning men and their health. We have already begun to glimpse the various ways that 'masculinity/masculinities' are understood and used within men's health policy and research. Yet, such conceptualizations are often implicit and hidden rather than explicit and central (though not in the later qualitative studies described above). There-fore, it is important now to understand explicitly how 'masculinity/mascu-linities' were conceptualized in this work for the purpose of exploring the empirical data presented in the chapters that follow.

Sociobiology, masculinity and health

At its most basic level, masculinity can be understood as the outward expressions of being biologically male. In this way, male (and female) beha-viours are accounted for through a form of genetic and/or biological deter-minism. The Y chromosome, testosterone and other hormonal influences, are seen as creating a drive towards particular behaviours in men – hunter (breadwinner), being territorial, sexual promiscuity – that are expressions of evolutionary mechanisms designed to ensure the survival of the species and the procreation of the strongest genetic pool. 'Society' has developed as a further evolutionary mechanism designed to restrain or channel the worst aspects of these behaviours or to develop positive expressions of them. As Clare (2001: 35) explains:

> For the sociobiologist, explanations of human behaviour can be located both within neurobiology and Darwinian evolutionary theory. Within such a schema, sex difference is easily explained and set in unyielding stone. The assertive, aggressive, thrusting, vigorous, urgent male serves evolution best by rushing around promiscuously impregnating as many females as he can.

Whilst strict adherence to this essentialist way of understanding sex differences in behaviour is rare, sociobiology continues to be a widely taught theory and to exert influence particularly in gendered representations in the popular press (Clatterbaugh 1990: 17; see also Clare 2001: Chapter 2; and Gough 2006).

Understanding masculinity in this way makes explanations for men's health relatively straight forward. Men's poorer health outcomes can be seen as stemming *directly* from a genetic predisposition and/or a hormonal drive that leads to predominantly destructive or damaging behaviours. There is certainly some evidence that the male genetic code does account for *some* differences in health outcomes between the sexes. For example, Kraemer (2000: 1609) states that 'the male foetus is at greater risk of death or damage from almost all obstetric catastrophes that can happen before birth' and that premature birth and stillbirth are more common amongst boys. This problem becomes compounded, he says, as developmental, conduct and oppositional disorders are all two to four times more common in boys. Likewise, recent evidence gathered by the Men's Health Forum (2004b) shows that men across Europe are more likely to develop and die from the ten most common cancers than women.

It is rare to find this way of conceptualizing masculinity as a single or sole explanation for the state of men's health but the following, humorously intended, comment from a general practitioner does suggest that it is often implicitly present in health professionals common-sense explanations of 'how men are':

> But will [men] abandon their traditional Saturday afternoon shin-kicking and beer-swilling in favour of a warm community centre, a slice of lentil bake and a group discussion on better foreskin hygiene? I doubt it. Aggression and foolhardiness are carried on the Y

chromosome and there's not a lot government or anyone else can do about it.

(Hammond 1994: 64)

Yet, the wide range of health inequalities that exist between the sexes, and health inequalities between men of different ethnic groups, social class and geographical regions cannot be accounted for in such a simplistic manner. In addition, seeing such differences as essential and fixed in this way leaves little or no possibility for change (see also Banks 2004: 156).

Role theory, masculinity and health

Psychological and sociological work has long questioned these biological-determinist explanations for human behaviour and an early alternative explanation for understanding human behaviour in modern society, including the differentiation of behaviours between the sexes, is that of 'role theory' mentioned briefly in the previous section. The basic assumption in role theory is that social expectations about a person's status in society produces conformity to a given role and its related sets of functions (neighbour, father, doctor, etc.). Fulfilment of these roles is encouraged through a range of implicit or explicit rewards and sanctions that are brought to bear in order to facilitate conformity (see Parsons 1964: Chapter 5). However, difficulties emerge when particular social roles will not or cannot be fulfilled. For example, society may expect that one of men's roles is to be a breadwinner and economic provider for his family and, even in the era of the 'new man', the relationship of paid employment to male identity remains strong (Haywood and Mac an Ghaill 2003: Chapter 1). If this view becomes internalized by an individual man who then becomes unemployed the result will be what Joseph Pleck terms sex role strain (Pleck 1981) or more recently male gender role strain (Pleck 1995). Thus, the greater the internalization of cultural norms of masculinity roles for an individual, which is what Pleck's psychological scales discussed earlier aim to measure, the greater the role strain experienced when these 'norms' cannot be lived up to.

This model is usually translated into health rhetoric in two ways that create a double bind for men. Firstly, there is the idea that traditional male roles themselves are detrimental to health; long hours, pressure to succeed, risk taking, and the stress related to these, can create psychological and (in some cases) ultimately physical ill health. Secondly, that failure to live up to these high-pressure roles and expectations can itself create pressures and strains that can result in feelings of failure, stress and related health symptoms. As one health journalist writes: 'It's hard being a man. You die younger and you're ill more often. But if you don't do the things that make you ill or have the potential to kill you, you're not considered a man' (Hobbs 1995: 14).

The idea of understanding masculinity through sex-role theory, and the development of psychological measures of masculinity to analyse this, has come under a great deal of criticism, mainly from sociologists. The criticisms are threefold. Firstly, it is said to lack sufficient historical perspective and therefore understanding of change. People are presented as empty vessels at birth that are socialized, or not, into particular ways of being (such as 'masculine') and within this framework: 'Change is always something that *happens to* sex roles, that impinges on them ... Sex-role theory cannot grasp change as a dialectic arising within gender relations themselves' (Carrigan et al. 1985: 578).

Secondly, and linked to the above, they are said to fail to address issues of power relations between men and women: 'The complex dynamics of gender identity, at both the social and the individual level, disappear in sex-role theory, as abstract opinions about "difference" replace the concrete, changing power relations between men and women' (Segal 1997: 69).

The third criticism often raised against sex-role theory is that it fails to *adequately* separate biological sex and gender. In this sense, as with the sociobiological explanations, it remains an essentialist way of thinking, one that creates rigid and fixed views about sex/gender differences. As Connell (1995: 26) states 'Sex roles are defined as reciprocal; polarization is a necessary part of the concept'. This being the case, it becomes clear to see how it is difficult to explore gender relations when they are presented as opposite ends of a continuum; that is as sex differences. This polarization also encourages a focus on differences rather than congruency and in this way helps obscure other important issues of identity such as class and race (Connell 1995: 27).

Postmodern views on masculinity

In response to recognizing these limitations within a role theory approach, Gutterman (1994) and Petersen (1998), amongst others, have specifically begun to explore the meaning of 'masculinity' within the postmodern context. They have drawn on the work of Judith Butler (1993), and other postmodernist writers on gender, to question the notion of 'masculinity' as a coherent concept. Unusually, an account of this approach to understanding masculinity in regard to health can be found in an article in the *British Medical Journal*:

> Postmodern theory ... breaks loose of any given definitions of those uncertain 'things' called sex and gender. We live in kaleidoscopes of fragmented and differing realities. A man may cry in one encounter and stoically withdraw in another, or do both. He may hold his teddy bear for comfort while refusing psychotropic drugs for fear of losing control ... Alternative theories of masculinity, as opposed to

'traditional' ones, help us to recognise when research is skewed and health care is sabotaged.

(Moynihan 1998: 1074)

Certainly the increasing number of comparative ethnographies of men (Cornwall and Lindisfarne 1994) and various situated accounts of men's lives (Jackson 1990; Kimmel and Messner 1998) speak of the numerous different experiences that constitute 'masculinity' as something other than a unified identity.

For these reasons of disparity some, such as Coleman (1990), argue against the usefulness of theorizing 'masculinity'. He maintains that masculinity is theorized in much sociological writing only in order to make causal links between social structures and masculine behaviour(s). As discussed earlier, to carry out empirical work on how male behaviours are created and sustained by social structures it is necessary to operationalize (and therefore theorize) the concept 'masculinity' that becomes a generic term for the 'doings of men'. This he suggests is folly. Using 'masculinity' as a way of 'rendering the doings of men visible and analysable' should not be necessary for sociologists. It is not their role to 'discover what is hidden or unknown and adumbrate it in theory' but rather to provide a 'perspicuous representation [of] what lies before us'. The work of sociology should not be about theorizing masculinity but attending to its 'occasions of use' (Coleman 1990: 193, 198). Yet, I would argue that it is precisely the need to illuminate that which is hidden that makes problematizing men by the use of a theoretical framework (masculinity/masculinities) so important. It is by *not* problematizing the category of 'male' in the research process that the 'doings of men' remain invisible and kept apart from critical scrutiny (Morgan 1981, 1992; Hearn and Morgan 1990: 7; Kimmel 1990). Postmodern approaches then, rather than being radical may, in practice, maintain the status quo by failing to theorize masculinity/masculinities as anything other than fragmented, incoherent and shifting concepts. Fear of using dualisms or 'categorizing' people and seeing 'power' only as a dispersed entity compound this problem in such approaches and can lead to a situation that fails to illuminate exactly that which then remains hidden; male privilege.

Clatterbaugh (1998) has also questioned the coherence of masculinity/ masculinities. He suggests that men's identities are too diverse for the term 'masculinity' to be of use and goes further to state that even if we use the term 'masculinities' to represent this diversity, it remains unclear what constitutes the component parts of this plural and who or how are people assigned to these component parts. He suggests a return to talking about 'men' as a way of reopening debates about men's position of domination in social institutions (and how this should be addressed), men's violence (and how this needs to be recognized and changed by men) as well as recognizing men's real yet different lived experiences. He specifically critiques postmodernist approaches for their inability to speak in language that can be clearly understood by men in society today and for advocating social change without 'any justification for that change' or, I would add, the direction that change should take apart from further deconstructions (see, for example, the concluding chapter in Haywood and Mac An Ghaill 2003).

A relational model of masculinity and health

It seems that an adequate theory of masculinity has to recognize the diversity of identity and difference among men and their health. Yet it also needs to retain a focus on the differential power relations between men and women, and between different groups of men, and how these both create, and are created and sustained, through social structures. In short, it has to take into account issues of agency and structure and recognize these as also having a cyclical relationship; that is, whilst individual actions might be constrained to a greater or lesser extent within social structures, social structures nevertheless are contingent on individuals' actions for their reproduction. Masculinity/masculinities need to be theorized in a way that embraces what Ginsburg (1992) has termed 'structured diversity'; that is, a model that can accept diversity amongst individuals yet continues to locate specifically where power operates both within groups of individuals and through societal structures.

Recently, some writers on gender and health (for example, Carpenter 2000) have suggested that a more coherent framework for understanding gender, masculinity (or more accurately masculinities) and its relationship to health, is that provided by Connell (1987, 1995, 2000). First and foremost, Connell's is a relational model; that is, gender is seen as being about sets of relations between men and women, but also relations *between* men and *between* women. Masculinities are a part of, and not distinct from, this larger system of relations that Connell terms the 'gender order'. Thinking about it in this way 'gives us a way of understanding the different dimensions or structures of gender, the relation between bodies and society, and the patterning or configuration of gender' (Connell 2000: 24).

Connell (1995) suggests that the relational patterning of masculinities in the current Western gender order consists of hegemonic, subordinated, marginalized and complicit masculinities. Table 1.2 summarizes Connell's work on this patterning, highlighting the key features of each aspect of masculinity within the gender order.

In order not to oversimplify this process and lead to a situation where we think there is *a* gay masculinity, *a* black masculinity, and so forth, and 'collapse into a character typology', Connell (1995: 76) again reinforces the need to maintain a focus on relational issues. He outlines how masculinities

Table 1.2   The patterning of contemporary masculinity (Connell 1995)

Hegemonic masculinity	'Hegemony' refers to the cultural dynamic by which a group claims and sustains a leading position in social life. Hegemonic masculinity is the configuration of practice that embodies the currently accepted answer to the problem of the legitimacy of patriarchy, which guarantees the dominant position of men. Hegemony is usually established through a correspondence between cultural ideals (such as exemplars in film like Sylvester Stallone) and collective institutional power. So, for example, we can talk of the health service as being a 'masculine' structure (Davies 1995).
Subordinated masculinity	In clarifying what constitutes hegemonic masculinity it is clear that other expressions of masculinity must be subordinate to this 'leading' position. Gay masculinity is perhaps the most conspicuous example of this and Connell makes it clear that the subordination is not just about cultural stigmatization but is also about material practices. Thus gay men often encounter cultural exclusion, abuse, violence and economic discrimination.
Marginalized masculinity	In addition to being subordinated to the 'leading' position, some expressions become marginalized from this position. There may be no direct, overt threat or attempt to exclude some expressions of masculinity (unlike gay masculinity) but they nevertheless become marginalized from full participation in society by material practices. Such a situation may arise for men with a physical impairment.
Complicit masculinity	Few men meet the normative standards of hegemonic masculinity, yet this does not stop these men benefiting from the general effect of this hegemony. The majority of men gain from the overall effect of the subordination of women and the subordination and marginalization of some men (as above) and thus share in what Connell terms the patriarchal dividend. This Connell terms complicit masculinity.

develop not as isolated acts but rather as actions configured in larger units that may be referred to as *configurations of gender practice*. In turn, these configurations also interact with other areas of social practice such as race, class, sexuality, and disability. Such configurations of gender practice are 'generated in particular situations in a changing structure of relationships' (Connell 1995: 81) and will inevitably include health practices, or practices that influence health status.

In this way, configurations of gender practice can be understood as recognized habitual practices that are open to change in new or differing circumstances. This allows masculinities to be understood as being historically contingent but not essentially determined (either by biology or processes of socialization) and as being fluid but hierarchical with dominant configurations acting collectively, becoming incorporated into the social structures of societies and thus replicating themselves. This process of inculcation into the social fabric occurs at both a representational and a material level at the expense of other configurations that become subordinated to and/or marginalized from the hegemonic forms. Configurations of practice that are complicit with this process may become necessary or desirable in gaining representational and thereby material privilege but also serve to replicate current gender hierarchies.

Summary

Current concerns and debates around the health of men have stemmed from several distinct but related areas including epidemiological data, trying to understand men's health 'behaviours' and situating these within the wider social context. The epidemiological patterning of male mortality and recent increases in rates of male specific morbidity has raised questions about how/why such patterning exists and how best it can be addressed. These concerns have been recognized at national government level within the UK, at least rhetorically, and attempts at strategic intervention to address male mortality have developed intermittently at local and regional levels since the early 1980s. However, the nature and amount of strategic intervention has varied greatly geographically – as has the level of support for various initiatives and the wider policy frameworks within which they sit. These shifting policy and policy implementation agendas have, in turn, influenced the ability, at a local level, for innovative initiatives not only to emerge but more importantly to be sustainable even when the will is there to develop health work aimed at men.

It is hardly surprising that there has been such *ad hoc* development of services given that the evidence base for considering what 'works' in terms of interventions to improve the health of men remains minimal or at least that the evidence that does exist has rarely been brought together.

Quantitative psychological and sociological research has provided insight into sex differences in health outcomes and related this to a range of social indicators and interestingly such work has often shown more similarity than difference between men and women. Likewise, survey work has identified some sex differences in the way that health is understood although, again, these are often less significant than might be expected. Qualitative research has illuminated why this might be the case as abstract notions about health, which men and women often share, become enacted out in different, gender specific ways in everyday life. More recent qualitative work has taken this notion further and begun specifically to look at the differing ways that 'masculinity' or 'masculinities' are presented, sustained or rejected in accounting for a range of health and health-related practices in various social settings.

All such policy, practice and research relies, either explicitly or implicitly, on particular ways of seeing how men are; particular understandings of what constitutes 'masculinity/masculinities'. The framework for understanding masculinities that influenced the collection and analysis of the empirical data that forms the rest of this book is predicated on a rejection of both socio-biological and 'role theory' explanations for understanding men and their social practices. Such essentialist explanations are overly deterministic and fail to account for men's own everyday understandings and experiences and also for the diverse nature of such social practices. Rather, masculinities here are understood as relational, as changing configurations of practice embedded in, and reproductive of, hierarchical social relations, rather than as a set of characteristics possessed (or not) by individual men. In this sense, masculinities are both the precursors to, and products of, intersubjective encounters. It is the aim of this book to examine new empirical data that consider how differing configurations of hierarchical masculinity practices both influence, and are influenced by, men's health practices.

Key points

- Present concerns about 'men's health' relate to mortality, morbidity and men's social practices (or 'behaviours').
- Despite increased policy recognition and innovations in practice little impact has been seen in men's health outcomes.
- Psychological research on the relationship of 'masculinity' to men's health practices/outcomes is often contradictory.
- Survey research has tended to show more similarities than difference in the way that men and women conceptualize health.
- Qualitative research has begun to show how, despite conceptualizing health in similar ways, it is enacted in gender specific ways by men and women in their daily lives.
- Sociobiological and 'role theory' explanations for men's health practices essentialize 'how men are' and fail to account for the diversity of practices amongst men.
- Understanding masculinities as hierarchical 'configurations of practice' that men move within and between provides a framework for exploring how and why men 'do' health differently in differing social contexts.

Key points for practice

- Understanding men's health practices as existing within wider sets of gendered social relations (rather than as being individual behaviours) allows us to explore how men's health interventions are not just about individual (male) change but are also about the potential for positive impact on families and communities.
- Previous qualitative research that explores how, when and why men draw on, and reject, male stereotypes is crucial to helping tailor more effective interventions.
- The way that health professionals conceptualize, either consciously or not, 'masculinity/masculinities' has implications for how they view men and how they think that men's health work should be approached.
- Essentialist ways of viewing 'masculinity' as a set of rigid (usually negative) traits, characteristics or drives can lead to professional inertia as the task of changing genetic/hormonal mechanisms or fixed intrapsychic structures seems, at best, hopeless and at worst impossible.
- Alternatively, understanding masculinities as configurations of social practices that men move between allows us to think about the opportunities that might occur to help encourage positive configurations in specific social contexts.

2 Conceptualizing health and well-being

Introduction

Whilst the sociological study of illness and the 'sick role' has a long and developing history, the sociological study of 'health' and 'well-being' has been slower to develop. As intonated in the previous chapter, this could be because health is taken for granted in everyday life and only becomes significant in its absence. Certainly, in early work on lay perspectives, a significant number of respondents identified health either as the absence of illness/disease or found it difficult to define, with health being seen as a 'normal', 'ordinary', daily state of being (for example, Blaxter 1990; Herzlich 1973; Williams 1983).

Yet lay understanding(s) of health and well-being are influenced by the meanings that health, illness and disease are ascribed in a society at given points in time. Thus, the historical movement from understanding illness and disease in spiritual terms, as sin, judgement or testing by God, to understanding them in terms of individual pathology, have also altered what constitutes 'health' and how it is to be understood. The medicalization of 'illness/disease' encourages this understanding of health as 'normal' and as the absence of this 'other', pathologized state.

Furthermore, despite this movement, concepts of 'health' continue to carry with them notions of morality and responsibility that are no longer mediated in spiritual terms but through notions of 'risk' 'probability' and 'susceptibility' (Lupton 1993). Crawford's (1984) empirical work highlights how issues of responsibility, control and release feature highly in such lay accounts. Likewise, Cornwell (1984) points out how people often gave a public, morally acceptable account concerning how they understood health and this differed from more private, socially integrated accounts, recounted through lived experiences and usually only elicited during further in-depth conversations.

It is the role that lay knowledge can play in providing understanding about this socially integrated nature of health practices that makes it so valuable. As has been argued in the introduction to this book, lay knowledge provides key information that is important in bridging the gap between issues of structure and agency in areas such as public health research (Popay and Williams 1996) and understanding inequalities in health (Popay et al. 1998;

Popay et al. 2003). Yet little work has been done to consider the important role of gender in creating and sustaining particular lay conceptualizations.

This chapter therefore begins by looking at how the men in this project articulated ideas about what constituted health, how they understood and defined the concept, how this relates to previous research on lay perceptions, and how such abstract definitions are gendered in nature. The following section then looks in detail at accounts of risk, responsibility, control and release which, whilst highly represented in the sociology of health and illness literature, and well-developed in health research with women (for example, Harding 1997; Howson 1998) have very rarely been looked at in terms of their gendered nature in health research with men.

What constitutes 'health'?

The conceptualizations of health for the men who took part in this study generally concurred with previous research on lay perceptions (see Hughner and Kleine 2004) and the more specific work undertaken on lay men's perceptions of health (Mullen 1993; Saltonstall 1993; Watson 2000) outlined briefly in the previous chapter. In addition, the concepts described were similar among all groups, although the specific emphasis differed at times between individual men and between the particular groups and these differences are outlined below.

Health as a 'non'-concept

It was clear that questions asking men to define health caused difficulties in knowing how to respond for some:

> SR: So if you were to think about what health meant to you, what would you say it was?
> Quinn: What do you mean?
> SR: If you were to try and define health.
> Quinn: Well, apart from me illness, I don't have any health problems. So I never think about it cause I'm fine apart from the illness.
>
> (Quinn DM2)

This could be because, as Bourdieu (1990) argues, the practices of everyday life, including health practices, are not wholly consciously organized but rather they are accomplished unthinkingly and routinely through what he terms 'practical consciousness'. This 'practical consciousness' develops from an individual's 'habitus', that is an acquired set of generative dispositions formed in the context of people's social locations. Yet part of what forms an individual's 'habitus' are the public metanarratives regarding what constitutes appropriate, gendered behaviour(s) or expressions of belief. In this regard, the idea, or expression, of not considering health may itself be linked in to notions of masculinity and gender. Blaxter (1990: 19) noted that three times as many men as women considered that health was a 'normal' state and, from the men's responses here, this does seem to be related in part to a wider public discourse that men are not, or should not be, interested in their health. As Quinn explains when asked if men think differently about health than women: 'Yeah, cause it's important to women innit, but blokes don't really bother about it. I mean speaking from my experience, like I say, I never think about it' (Quinn DM2). And from Martin: 'I think it's, it's not even an attitude, it's a non-attitude towards health. They [men] don't see it as a problem. I don't think they think that going out and having a binge on Friday night's a problem' (Martin CABS3).

Part of what constitutes being a (real) man is therefore about being unconcerned regarding notions of health, yet, such public expressions do not always relate to men's concrete health practices.

That men assumed or presumed health, took it for granted, and did not think about it, was also the commonest representation amongst health professionals. Again, this presumption was often specifically linked to aspects of male identity:

> I think men are under a great deal of pressure during their working life, and through fatherhood, to be fit and healthy and therefore to presume they are fit and healthy. And if you go for screening you are doubting that you're fit and healthy and I don't think men allow themselves the opportunity to doubt that.
>
> (Collette HP2)

In this sense, expressions of concepts regarding 'health' cross-cut and sometimes conflict with notions of male identity. There is a moral obligation to care for one's health; yet at the same time, to demonstrate masculinity, one must give at least public expression to non-concern with health; I term this the 'don't care/should care' dichotomy and shall return to it later in the chapter.

Health as functionality

The idea of health as being the absence of illness/disease was almost always linked to notions of health as being able to function: 'I class being healthy as being able to do things most other people, well people who aren't disabled, or that haven't got an illness, can do' (Gary GM3).

However, in contrast to the men in Watson's (2000) research, for only a very few of the men in this project was this idea of functioning *specifically* related to the fulfilling of the male 'role' of breadwinner/provider. Work by Riska (2002) suggests that medical/psychological discourses of male identity in relation to work have changed over the last 50 years. These changing discourses, from stressed out, 'Type A' executive, to a 'Hardy Man' who incorporates and works with stress as a motivator, may (she says) have been necessary to prepare men for changes in the division of labour and the need for more flexible working patterns in late capitalism.

Work was certainly cited regularly as something that contributed to men's physical and mental health and well-being and this contribution was seen as both positive and negative at different times. Yet this was not always discussed purely at a personal level. Several of the men were aware that changes in employment patterns, particularly the movement of more women into the workplace and concomitant increases in men's involvement in the domestic sphere, altered perceptions of work in society and this was generally heralded as a positive change:

> ...but going back to what you were saying, the attitudes are chan-
> ging now, especially I suppose with childcare. Men can get more
> paternity leave, so they see more of their kids, spending more time at
> home. I think the whole work ethos, apart from like these high-
> browed sort of sales jobs, is a bit more relaxed.
>
> (Francis, CABS1)

Being physically active, including activity at work, was seen as both a signifier of, and contributor to, health and well-being. In response to being asked about a time in their lives when they felt particularly healthy or well, answers nearly always included descriptions of actual activities. These included accounts of feats of physical fitness, work that they could previously perform but could not any longer, and being able to socialize, drink all night, and still be up early the next day. This relationship of activity to health is made explicit by Quinn: 'When I could run and that I suppose I felt healthier then because I ran and was active. Um, but as me legs got worse I slowed down and I suppose me health got a bit less because I wasn't active' (Quinn DM2).

Health in this sense becomes integrally linked to functionality such that loss of function denotes loss of health. Even though, as we saw previously, Quinn considers himself to have no health problems, he still links his loss of physical function to the concept of having a poorer health status. The hegemonic defining of masculinity through bodily function (Connell 1995: 45), through doing rather than being (Morgan 1992), makes this linking of health with functionality commonplace for many men. It demonstrates, as Saltonstall (1993: 10) suggests, that ideas about health are mediated through ideas about one's gendered identity and for men this usually entails the linking of health to the medium of action with the ability to function claiming paramount importance. In this way it is often the case that while function remains intact and taken for granted, health does also.

Whilst physical activity and functionality were important concepts that men used in regard to defining health, in contrast to previous studies,[1] 'health as fitness' appeared in only three of the direct definitions given by the men. However, when the men spoke about what had a positive effect on health and well-being, fitness/exercise were frequently mentioned. It seems there is a distinction between defining health *as* fitness/exercise and achieving health *through* fitness/exercise. If (hegemonic) masculinity is constructed, or performed, through 'doing' (Morgan 1992), then it is no surprise that being a 'healthy' male is characterized by optimum physical functioning achieved for some through fitness/exercise.

Health, the lifecourse and 'feeling'

Blaxter (1990: 30) has shown that lay perceptions about what constitutes 'health' change across the lifecourse. Recent work by McGowan (2002) suggests that when looking back at health over the lifecourse, it is common for men to reflect on a time when they were younger and they felt that the body was in 'peak condition'. This was certainly reflected in the findings of this study with 15 of the 20 men choosing this type of description when asked about a time when they felt particularly healthy or well:

> When I lived in Bahrain that was my peak shall we say. There's a picture of me [...] I titled it 'Tanned God', beautiful tan, it was the time of my life I felt the best. I felt fabulous 'cause we used to go swimming in beautiful warm, clear, blue sea virtually everyday.'
>
> (Bob, CABS6)

For those who described the present as a time when they were healthy or well, this was also often related to a concept of health as 'feeling' and seems to be a concept different from that captured by much previous work on lay perceptions.[2] For these men this 'feeling' was not an abstract concept but was formed through current circumstances. So for Owen, the present feeling of being healthy is linked to an anticipated career change, giving up work, spending more time with his young family and having the time to commence more physical activity. For Larry current success in developing his own business generated these present feelings of health or well-being: 'I think this branch, when I've opened the shop, is where I've felt best, physical and mental at my best [...] I tell you what, I didn't even feel this healthy before I had diabetes, you know what I mean. So I think now I'm at my healthiest. (Larry, CABS4)

Likewise, for Peter the coming together over the last two years of the birth of twins following IVF treatment, recent positive change of job, and the consistent support of a loving wife, led him to say: 'I feel extremely healthy and well at the moment. For the past two years I haven't had any pressures in my life' (Peter, DM1).

Thus, although Owen could be said to be linking health to fitness, Larry to work, and Peter to positive life changes, it is the *feeling* generated from having the time to participate in fitness, achieving at work or having children and a successful marriage, that constitutes what is 'healthy' in their narratives. In this sense, 'health' may be related to feelings of existential or onto-logical security and this is explored further in Chapter 4. Understanding health in this way links with other narratives suggesting that mental health or emotional well-being was an integral part of being 'healthy' and could not be separated from physical well-being, as Neil succinctly puts it when asked to define health: 'Well-being state of body and mind' (Neil GM5).

Victor Seidler (1994) suggests that, within the present Enlightenment vision of modernity, masculinity is premised upon the separation of the mind and body, what has become known as Cartesian dualism. In particular, he pays attention to how the mind came to be valued above the body and how men became associated with the mind and thereby with reason, and women with the body and thereby with nature and emotionality. Yet, for these men, whilst the concepts of mental and physical health were often rhetorically separated, they tended to be more integrated when concrete experiences were being recounted:

> I have problems with my legs with the MS [Multiple Sclerosis] and it [yoga] keeps them supple, helps you focus your mind as well. Sometimes, you get so much happening to you in a day, so much input, it's difficult for your brain to sort of focus it all into a steady stream, to analyse it, it's just bombarding.
>
> (Bob, CABS6)

This linking of the need for mental relaxation and the physical benefit it confers with regard to his MS is no coincidence and Bob makes the same link during the second interview:

> I have actually done quite a bit of meditating just recently because it's my leg again. But I've been meditating, staying calm so that I can process everything that is happening around me [...] Stress and MS don't go well together.
>
> (Bob, CABS6)

Having said this, the separation of the mental from the physical can remain important for men when seeking help for health issues and this is also con-sidered further in Chapter 4.

For other men, understanding health as 'feeling' was linked strongly to body image and 'looking good' and this is discussed in more detail in the following chapter. It is worth noting here though that whilst commentators have identified the part that consumer culture plays in connecting notions of *looking good* to those of *being healthy* (for example, Shilling 1993), previous research on lay perceptions of health has suggested that this view is less common amongst men (Blaxter 1990: 24; Saltonstall 1993). But, in line with previous work specifically on lay men's perceptions (Mullen 1993; Watson 2000), work here suggests that health can be synonymous with looking good for some men.

One man could not recall a time when he had felt healthy or well when asked: 'Not really no. I just always feel the same unless I'm in more pain than usual. I've never felt really ... No, as far as I can remember I've never felt like on top of the world type of thing' (Quinn DM2). It seems highly likely that this lack of *feeling* healthy for Quinn is again rooted in both physical and social circumstances. Life has presented Quinn with a series of struggles and challenges from spending part of his childhood in care to his increasing physical impairment from a progressive, degenerative disease. Yet, his presentation is far from that of victim. On the contrary, narratives about 'just getting on with life' and feeling impatient with disabled friends who feel sorry for themselves, constituted a large part of his interview narratives. And, despite not *feeling* healthy, he frequently presents himself as having no health problems and goes so far as to say: 'I'm quite healthy, not because I keep myself fit, I'm just like that for some reason. Maybe it's nature compensating for the illness, I don't know, I've had mine [impairment] all me life and I've never really had a day of sickness' (Quinn, DM2).

Viewing differently

For one group of men interviewed, the gay men, despite the incorporation of the above elements within their narratives, all saw health through a particular lens: that of sexual health and risk. Six out of the seven directly incorporated sexual health and/or risk rhetoric into their definitions of health. As Wayne says when asked to define health: 'Being safe. Obviously, you know, in a sexually liberated country as England is I think ... hygiene you know is foremost because the rise of STDs is phenomenal' (Wayne, GM6).

That gay men see health through such a lens is not surprising given that, as Hart and Flowers (2001: 226) point out, they have been 'defined medically in terms of what they do in bed'. This powerful discourse, constructing gay male health as being synonymous with sexual health, is then combined with the fact that many of the gay men interviewed had previously lost friends through HIV/AIDS and two were HIV positive: 'Things have changed a lot from what it was when it [HIV/AIDS] first started. I can remember when I was going to a funeral virtually every week. I haven't been to a good funeral now for over a year!' (Edward, GM2).

A powerful interplay exists between the strong public discourse connecting gay health to sexual health and the concrete experiences that these gay men have had of losing friends to HIV/AIDS. This combination acts to make a sexual health script predominant for gay men when considering health issues, although this is not the sole public discourse available to gay men and other narratives about gay men drinking, smoking and taking more drugs were also prevalent. Together, such narratives and experiences lead to ideas about risk and morality being given primacy in discussions with gay men about health. This is discussed further shortly.

In concluding this section, it needs to be highlighted that in reading the interview accounts in full, the conceptualizations of health and well-being outlined above were not as disparate as they have been presented. Indeed most interviews comprised several of the elements discussed, showing a complex interplay between the different conceptualizations:

> Um, you know feeling healthy in yourself. Some people prefer being healthy in as much as they feel a good weight, prefer doing sport to keep themselves healthy, dose themselves up with multi-vits and make sure they're not run down, or if they look good it feels healthy.
> (Francis, CABS1)

It is also clear that abstract definitions of health do not come readily to the men. The health professionals believed that this indicated a lack of concern for health, but the men's own narratives suggest that it is because health is integrally tied to the ability to function in daily life, not something that can be abstracted out. In turn, positive accounts of daily life lead to a 'feeling' of being healthy. In this way health, as physicality and emotionality, can begin to be distinguished as a truly and fully embodied concept and this is examined in more detail in the following two chapters.

Issues of risk, responsibility, control and release

As highlighted in the introduction to this chapter, abstract notions about health are often intertwined with aspects of morality. Whilst the issue of where responsibility for 'health' lies remains highly politically contested, risks to health, and the ability to control such risks, have undoubtedly become the new *raison d'être* of health promotion services and professionals. This section explores how risk, responsibility, and the associated notions of control and release, whilst often discussed in gender neutral terms, are actually played out, and played with, at the intersection of health and (gendered) identity.

The particulars of control and release

It is clear that health carried moral connotations for the men being presented in its simplest form as what one should or should not do:

SR: What does health mean to you?
Neil: Er, it does mean a lot, but I don't tend to it as much as what I should do.

(Neil, GM5)

Using a Foucauldian framework, writers such as Armstrong (1983, 1995) and Petersen and Lupton (1996) have suggested that government, working with and through the medical profession, both generates and uses such moral discourses around health as part of a wider political function; namely surveillance and regulation.

The ultimate regulation, as Foucault (1980: 155) suggests, is achieved through self-surveillance and this is why incorporation of moral accounts of health into individual identities becomes so important. It is when this incorporation is achieved that expressions of control by individuals in relation to health become significant as recognizing one's limits becomes representative of correct moral behaviour: 'Generally, like smoking, drinking, drugs, you know, if your doin' it then obviously you should know what your limit is' (David, GM1).

Some writers (Petersen and Lupton 1996; Higgs 1998) have suggested that this individualization of surveillance represents part of a wider move in social policy to shift responsibility for health (and other areas) onto the individual. Primacy is given to the role of agency rather than structure in determining health outcomes and the role of the state becomes one of providing information on which individuals can choose (or not) to act and in providing rewards or sanctions to encourage 'correct' individual lifestyle choices.

Within this Foucauldian framework, transgression of these suggested boundaries, reluctance/refusal to exert self-control, becomes reinterpreted as an act of subversion, or resistance, and health becomes a political arena wherein dominant discourses, as signifiers of authority, are challenged. However, such a model was not reaffirmed by the empirical data from this research. There were no examples of transgressing boundaries as a challenge to authoritative control being present in the interviews.[3]

Crawford (1984, 2000) proposes an alternative explanatory model regarding issues of control *and release*. He affirms that modern medicine has extended surveillance through the moralizing rhetoric of health promotion, that this has been internalized by individuals, and is used as a way of managing and maintaining 'healthy producers'; that is, as a form of regulation. Yet, he also recognizes that capitalism in late modernity also requires the same individuals to be consumers, an ideal that has become synonymous with 'fun, immediate gratification, and a propensity to exceed limits' (Crawford 2000: 222). In this sense, 'a little bit of what you fancy does you good'; release from control becomes constructed as healthy *in itself*. Strict adherence to bodily disciplinary regimes and lifestyles has to be offset by release, pleasure, often actively constructed in opposition to a 'healthy life-style', in order to achieve a 'healthy balance'. This interplay of control and release, played out in the health arena amongst other areas, is seen as a system requirement in late capitalism and creates an impossible task for health promotion in managing this ambivalent relationship.[4]

Martin provides an example of how this tension is managed through an understanding of health as balance, or as life needing all things in moderation:

> I do keep fit. Um don't drink too much, don't smoke too much, well I probably do at times [laughs]. Watching what I eat to a certain extent, eating fruit and vegetables. Um, so keeping fit, eating healthily and not living life in too much of an excess.
>
> (Martin, CABS3)

and after describing a recent hangover following a night out with friends:

> *Martin:* Generally I don't drink too much, I don't really smoke so I guess that's the worst kind of binge drinking going out the odd Friday and getting plastered, but . . .
>
> *SR:* And would you say actually going out and doing that could be seen as healthy?
>
> *Martin:* No. Well I don't know, I guess it is. Being happy is practically as much a cure for anything, positive mental attitude I guess can work wonders. Having a good night out, a good few social drinks, so I guess it's the feel-good factor isn't it?
>
> (Martin, CABS3)

The rhetoric of balance and moderation was frequently invoked in this way as a means of trying to bring together the need for control and the desire for release in terms of health practices and this suggests that Crawford's model has more resonance with the men's experiences. Some men even went as far as recognizing this tension as an inherent part of modern life and driven by consumerism:

> I eat healthy food generally and I cheat now and again. Alcohol's bad for you, but we all drink, mostly everyone I know likes a drink, cause it's good for you, it actually cheers you up [. . .] We've got like this throw-away society and I think people's perceptions are changing, everybody wants everything yesterday. People want to gain as much as possible materialistically, physically and emotionally. And that's

it, get fit one day, get drunk the next, buy the best house in the country the day after you know, and that's a full life.

(Dan, CABS7)

The multiplicity of risk

This moralizing of health, which leads to consideration of issues of control and release, is mediated through ideas about risk. 'Healthy citizens' are those who recognize, and limit (and transgress?) risks both to themselves and others; this is part of a wider duty to achieve and maintain good health (Petersen and Lupton 1996: Chapter 3).

Yet notions of 'citizenship', and therefore what constitutes risk, are themselves gendered. In work on masculinity and health, men are represented at various times as both 'risk takers' (in terms of fast driving, excessive drinking, smoking, violence) and those 'at risk' (in terms of high mortality rates, particularly amongst young men) and these two risk rhetorics are often combined to form a circle of explanation regarding men's health. That is to say the 'risk taking' is, at least in part, seen as responsible for the mortality/ morbidity that situates them as 'at risk'. There were strong narratives, particularly from the health professionals, that men were often careless with regard to the risks they took with their health. This carelessness being linked to peer group pressure and the need to perform a 'macho' style of male behaviour:

> It's just an assumption of health really. You know, you can drink, you can eat, you can smoke and do all these things. It's all an ado-lescent sort of attitude really, a cavalier attitude to their health really, you know, sort of 'macho', one of the boys.

(Collette HP2)

Immaturity, or childishness, was rhetoric also used by some of the men themselves to describe or explain both risk-taking behaviour and lack of care over health concerns.

Lyons and Willott (1999: 293ff) have found this discourse, of 'man as infant' (amongst other discourses) in their analysis of representations of men's health in women's magazines and suggest it serves the purpose of resolving the contradiction between 'men being opposed to health and women as responsible [for health]'. They point to how such notions represent a switch in gendered representations as men become associated with irra-tional, emotional (projected as childish) responses and women with a dominant, rational, active self. Yet gendered identity is complex and is formed and reformed in relation to varied and contradictory discourses and this is particularly the case for issues around masculinity and risk. How this tension between male lack of care and female responsibility for health impacts on men's engagement with health services is discussed further in Chapter 5.

Others suggest that to be a good male citizen is to invite in, rather than avoid, risk, and health then becomes subsumed under the need to form (or express) one's masculine identity in this way (Petersen and Lupton 1996: 80*ff*). Certainly the men were all aware of this 'macho' aspect of male identity but nearly all distanced themselves from it in direct discussion: '... men have been taught from a child that you have this "you're a man, you're supposed to be big and nothing bothers you" and all that, but it's not true, it's not true' (Frank, DM6).

In order to unpack these emerging issues around risk further, a question asking if the men could describe a time when they had deliberately put their health at risk was asked during second interviews. The replies from some of the men seem to crystallize the significant role that control/release plays as a moralizing discourse not just for health but also in the construction/ expression of male identity:

> Nothing instantly springs to mind, obviously driving too fast, smoking too many fags, drinking too much beer, but it's not what I see as putting myself at risk, it's not like playing chicken or anything like that with an oncoming car. So, everything I've done is I guess measured and controlled within what I think are safety sort of parameters really. So I don't generally take too big a risk.
>
> (Martin, CABS3)

This issue of risk control was also present for Frank and linked to a conversation about masculinity and risk:

> Just the way I drive a car and everything, I drive as if I'm in the TT races, that's part of posing. I don't do it when she's [wife] in the car, she'd kill me. Even if I was on my own with the kids, I wouldn't do it. I don't mind putting myself at risk but I wouldn't do it to me kids. No. Because I think I'm in control of the car so if I end up killing meself it's my fault you know, but they're innocent, so yeah.
>
> (Frank, DM6)

In this sense, for most of the men, risk is invited in, but not in an unmeasured way. Connell (1995: 54*ff*) suggests that (hegemonic) masculinity is framed, in part, through a combination of force and skill and accounts such as the two above suggest that 'risk' activity was often engaged in in these terms: as a test of force and/or skill to control extremes (of drinking, driving, sporting activities). This mirrors the notion of 'edgework' proposed by Collison (1996) who described how young male offenders mobilized notions of 'risky' activities they had been involved in, 'living on the edge', as a means of performing dominant masculinity, although the accounts here do not *directly* replicate the notion of 'edgework' as understood by Collinson. He relates 'edgework' to a need to transcend the banality of everyday existence for the young men in his research. The understanding of 'edgework' here is different, as it can also represent part of an 'ordinary', regular part of being male, or demonstrating hegemonic masculinity *in* daily life, not solely as a transcendence of it. It seems that this 'edge' is representative of a path between control and release that must be walked to reach or maintain (hegemonic) male identity. Yet, as we shall see shortly, movement away from the edge may itself become the requirement of good (male) citizenship when issues of responsibility also have to be considered at certain stages of the lifecourse. For the disabled men, this 'edge' can have both symbolic and concrete meaning:

> I probably do put me health at risk too many times cause I'm always doing, *I'm always on the edge, I'm always doing summit what I'm close to tipping over.* Like I go fishing and I'll fish about an inch from the edge and its like a ten foot drop.
>
> (Ron, DM4, emphasis added)

The physical edge of the lake, the proximity to 'tipping over' both literally and metaphorically, becomes a place where Ron courts danger and demonstrates his masculinity through courage and control of his wheelchair. In this sense, the risk involved is not only the very real physical risk of falling in the lake, and possibly drowning, but potential embarrassment through loss of control. Whilst Ron does not specify which risk he is identifying here, the rest of his interview narratives indicate that both represent threats to his health and well-being. For all the disabled men, the question about putting themselves at risk incorporated rhetoric about bodily vulnerability related to their particular impairment. In this sense risk becomes more overtly embodied for these men and this is discussed in more detail in the following chapter.

Risk was also related to particular aspects of the lifecourse, when transgression, as Lupton (1999: 159) has pointed out, is actually an expected part of normal, young (male) behaviour:

> When I was younger, I lived with a pal of mine in a flat for six months. And we probably took it to the extreme in most things at that time, drinking, eating, living in grime as it were, you know, staying up till the sun came up. All that normal stuff, I don't think I'm any different than most.
>
> (Owen, CABS5)

The men did not restrict such behaviour at this stage of the lifecourse to men and were acutely aware of changing practices and discourses about young women's increasing engagement in activities such as drinking, smoking, violence and extreme sports.

This association of 'risk taking' with young (male) behaviour was also something mentioned by some of the health professionals:

> Men of that age [25–40 years] are aware of issues around how much they should be drinking, that they shouldn't be smoking, what their diet ought to be, but it's not ranked as something that's particularly important to them. I think that's because its not something that will impinge on them until a much later stage in their life.
>
> (John, HP3)

For other health professionals the strong discourse of men as 'risk takers' was brandished without regard to lifecourse and this has obvious implications for the relationship between men and health professionals.

Risk versus risk

Discussions about masculinity and risk in the health literature often take place in a void, abstracted from other aspects of daily existence and unlinked to empirical data. In reality, for the men in this research, 'risky' lifestyle behaviour was very much socially integrated and often engaged in to offset other practices also perceived as 'risky' in health terms. This links in with Carter's work on masculinity and risk and his recognition that: 'Discourses of masculinity often classify risks into two dimensions; the taking of some and avoiding of others. Masculine identity becomes a complex negotiation between these two risk dimensions' (Carter 1993: 158). Smoking seemed to provide a particular example of this for three of the men and was perhaps most clearly expressed in Hugh's interviews, as the following lengthy extracts show:

> *SR:* You know, like the smoking and drinking do you see those as like a release?
>
> *Hugh:* Oh yeah. Nearly every chef I know smokes. Nearly every chef I know cause its such a stressful job and its just cause you don't get breaks as well. I can do like 12 hours without a break, so it's just, I'll sit down for 5 minutes, have a fag and calm meself down and everything. I mean you might not smoke a full cigarette, but having it lit and just sitting, you know it just gives a chance to sit down for 5 minutes.
>
> *SR:* Yeah, and so in a way that in itself could actually be seen as being healthy?
>
> *Hugh:* Its not meant to be healthy, is it? But to me it's my form of release from the pressure of my job. It's like a drink. I always have a pint after work. As soon as I finish me work and everything, sit down and have

a drink before I come home. To try and calm meself down a bit before I actually get home and then I'll probably have another can or two cans when I get in. They're like releases of stress for me you know part of cooling down, chilling out.

[. . .]

Hugh: Its like I said on the last one [interview] with me smoking. I do enjoy a cigarette you know, cause its one form for me ... how I'd cope without them I don't know. Like me friend who works with me. He's just had a triple bypass you know. He used to smoke and everything and he got warned about it, he had an heart attack and he didn't stop and he's carried on. So you know it does put things in me mind ... It's the second chef I've known that's had to go through this. I know I should give up smoking and that for the kiddies but its just that I don't know how I'd cope, you know.

SR: With the mental side of things?

Hugh: Yeah, without it.

Hugh takes his work very seriously and narratives about the importance of not phoning in sick, never having had a day off work, and the restaurant trading off his name, are prevalent in the interviews. Yet he attaches a high stress level to the job and sees smoking, and having a few drinks after work, as a means of reducing the stress and thereby the risk to his health posed by stress, whilst recognizing that these activities in themselves pose a risk to his health. Thus, in line with Graham's (1987) research into women's smoking, the empirical data here also suggest that specific 'unhealthy' practices (for Hugh, smoking and high alcohol intake) are engaged in as a means of coping with real, material pressures of everyday life that are experienced as presenting 'risks' to health and well-being.

Likewise, for Bob, 'risky' behaviour was engaged in during time in the army to avoid another very real risk posed by not engaging in these practices: the risk of non-inclusion/acceptance. After explaining the contrast between the physical fitness regime and the excessive smoking and drinking he engaged in during this time he goes on to explain:

> You're in a group of 30 people and they're all trying to be the 'macho' man, the Alpha male. And you think 'Oh', you don't want to go against the grain cause then you're automatically picked on. So you're 'Go on, I'll have that cigarette, and I'll have that one extra beer.' [. . .] If you're not in this streamlined group, you're shunned, you just don't fit, and if you don't fit then ...

> (Bob, CABS6)

This is not 'macho posturing' for the sake of it and such views on the potential risks attached to non-acceptance, and the role of smoking, drinking and so forth in gaining acceptance in the armed forces, was supported by narratives in Hugh's interviews and has been noted in previous critical autobiographical work by Morgan (1987). These accounts suggest that notions of 'risk' (and the control of risks) are mobilized in different ways at different times in the construction of male identity, the process of which is ongoing and at times is brought into explicit focus. For Peter the sudden experience of severe physical impairment at the age of 20 necessitated a reconsideration of identity and specifically male identity. This (re)construction required engaging in 'risky' behaviour in order to gain acceptance and specifically acceptance as a man:

> I've been out with girls, I think I went though a stage when I first broke me back of proving my manhood, I was a right git towards women, I used to have one after the other. I was trying to prove me manhood again, that I still had it.
>
> (Peter, DM1)

> I suppose when I first moved back I got in with a crowd who took drugs basically and I went with the crowd. Because of my medical condition I really could have caused myself some damage I suppose. I was trying to fit in [...] I suppose that was about getting respect because I'm associated with this person who is, or was, one of the biggest dealers in this area.
>
> (Peter, DM1)

A simplistic model of explanation in relation to risk taking and male identity, that of inviting risk in, fails to do justice to the complexity of the issues of control, release and identity formation for these men. The 'risks' taken by Peter, being sexually promiscuous and taking drugs, would have quite a different meaning for women, possibly resulting in social isolation or non-acceptance, rather than as a means of being accepted. 'Risk' in this sense is not about probability, the chance of an event happening, but is integrated, woven, into the gendered fabric of society's expectations.

The externalizing of risk

Sociological critiques of health promotion have pointed out that, despite a rhetoric of the need for structural change, most health promotion activity remains at the level of the individual, making it almost synonymous with lifestyle choices regarding eating, smoking, exercise and so forth (Nettleton and Bunton 1995: 44). This individualization fails to take into account not only the weighing of risks and the interaction of health practices with the project of masculinity outlined above, but also the real threat, and management, of external risks encountered by the men in their everyday lives. Whilst all the men individualized the issue of risk when raised as a direct question, the more private accounts found in other narratives suggested that very real risks, beyond their control, existed alongside this and that these also had to be managed.

All the gay men gave occasions when they had engaged in unprotected sex as the main example of when they had deliberately put their health at risk. Yet the encountering of homophobia and the difficult decisions regarding 'coming out' described by these men all serve as examples of external risks to health and well-being that are rarely, if ever, addressed through health promotion. As Kieran explains when talking about 'coming out':

> All I can say is you've got to make sure you have back-up, a fall back position if you like, and that you are aware of what might happen. I mean, when I came out at work I had to decide whether I was happy in me job and whether I was happy not to progress any further. And I had to seriously consider that, yeah. Now if I worked in a factory full of fellers I might have thought differently.
>
> (Kieran, GM4)

Threats to one's health are not a simple matter of lifestyle choices. Notions of 'risk' do not stand alone, separate from other aspects of identity, but can actually occur as a result of an identity position. Kieran experienced the potential risk of loss of opportunities at work, and of physical violence, in declaring his sexuality. Connell (1995: 76*ff*) points out that it is through such real, material circumstances that hierarchies of masculinity become constructed, and some masculinities, such as gay masculinities, become subordinated to the hegemonic standards against which they are measured and found wanting. A further example of this is provided by Gary who felt obliged to keep his sexuality from his GP:

> I didn't tell him [previous GP] I was gay. At the time I was worried about insurance issues like I say and that sort of thing. It wasn't that I was scared of telling the doctor, it was just that I didn't want the information being used against me.
>
> (Gary, GM3)

Gary goes on, though, to contrast this with a later time, after he has been diagnosed HIV positive, when he felt the risk of disclosing his sexuality, this time to his dentist, was more important because of the potential benefit of his dentist being able to detect early signs of changes in immune system functioning.

These external risks were not restricted to the gay men and all the other men identified external risks in their private narratives. Also, the health professionals identified the risks posed externally by poverty to particular men, which was not surprising given the strong discourses around inequalities in health over the last two decades, although most professionals felt that working to correct such inequalities was beyond their ability or remit:

> I don't think we're born on a level playing field, I think the day a child comes into the world there's inequality [...] I think as health visitors we're very aware of that unfairness. I don't know how we address it, cause I think addressing it has to come from central government.
>
> (Collette, HP2)

It is clear then that 'risk' can be seen as relating to both external circumstances and individual choices and this brings us back to having to consider that the management of health risks can therefore be seen as having a moral element, usually discussed in terms of 'responsibility'.

Further issues of responsibility in health and well-being

That men's presentation as being 'unconcerned' about health may be related more to a dominant discourse about how men ought to behave rather than the private reality of men's lives, has been highlighted in the opening section of this chapter. As mentioned, many of the men and the health professionals felt that men, on the whole, did not consider health either at all or certainly not as a priority. Yet, when this rhetoric was invoked by the men, they frequently distanced themselves from personally being like that, suggesting that this was how *men were* but not necessarily how *they are*. This distancing can be seen as a way of resolving, or managing, two conflicting discourses: first, that 'real' men don't care about health and second, that the pursuit of health is a moral requirement for good citizenship: the 'don't care/should care' dichotomy.

Previous work (Backett and Davison 1995) has examined how lifecourse events impact on and influence lifestyle in relation to health practices. The taking on of individual responsibilities, particularly settling with a long-term partner and becoming a father, altered not only the way that men thought about health but their actual health practices and this will be considered in more detail in Chapter 4. In relation to issues of control, release and morality, it is necessary to look briefly at this area here. Owen explains the impact of fatherhood in discussions on health, lifestyle and risk:

> I do everything that normal people do which is why we drink, go out at weekends, we eat take-away's but we eat at home as well, we do

> everything a mixture. I can't think of any time that we've really done
> it to excess, especially not now I've got me daughter.
>
> (Owen, CABS5)

and

> It did change when [daughter] was born, you try and get as much
> sleep as you can, eat when you can, you've got to look after yourself
> cause you've got to be alert, ready, you know just in case.
>
> (Owen, CABS)

A need to exert self-control predominates over the desire for release at particular ages and stages of the lifecourse for the men, resulting in changes in health-related practices and this finding is supported by previous work on lay men and health (Mullen 1993; Watson 2000). This change in lifestyle seems to be due to two separate (but probably interrelated) moral elements that require emotional investment. First, it seems to be deontologically driven; that is, it is rule based. To be a good, dutiful, partner and father, as Owen suggests above, requires the limiting of excess in order to be alert and available to meet the needs of a dependant. Second, it seems to be teleologically driven; that is, driven by recourse to outcomes, in this case the desire to be there for the child as it grows older and therefore to live long enough to enjoy this. As Larry explains when asked if he feels it important to live a long life:

> It wasn't when I didn't have [his son]. But it is now, I want to enjoy
> him, I want him to know that he can enjoy me, you know. Let him
> know that I'll be here for him at every stage of the way basically. It's
> very important to me to know that he can see me anytime, talk to me
> about anything. I'll work my rocks off for him, you know what I
> mean? The business is his, the house is his, and everything I have is
> his, full stop.
>
> (Larry, CABS4)

This is more than just rhetoric for Larry who is diabetic and prior to getting married and becoming a father refused to inject insulin for over 18 months, due to a needle phobia. He now feels it sufficiently important to work through this phobia and consider other lifestyle choices in order to maximize his health and longevity for the sake of his son and his own desire to see him grow up.

The need to demonstrate hegemonic masculinity through 'edgework', treading a narrow path between control and release, takes on reduced significance as men move into stable partnerships, including gay partnerships, and fatherhood. Yet this does not necessarily represent a move away from hegemonic ideals. As Owen and Larry's narratives suggest, hegemonic ideals of taking control and being the material provider are drawn on to support this change in reducing the propensity towards excess. In this sense, what constitutes a hegemonic masculine ideal may alter through the lifecourse and the expectation to demonstrate 'edgework', a hegemonic ideal for younger or single men, shifts towards an ideal of 'controlling excess' when the responsibility of a stable relationship, and particularly fatherhood, are entered into. This process seems to be at least partly reversible and some propensity towards excess, particularly drinking and sexual promiscuity, returned for two of the men, Bob and Larry, who separated from their partners, one just before and one during the course of the fieldwork. Yet, their role as fathers did act to constrain their participation in other excesses or risks that had constituted part of their youth. This suggests that what constitutes hegemonic masculinity can vary depending on the particular social site or period. Wetherell and Edley (1999) identify the importance of the presentation of an 'ordinary', non-heroic masculinity in the (re)production of hegemonic masculinity. The men's narratives here seem to support this and suggest that such 'ordinary' masculinity is sustained through recourse to hegemonic norms of 'responsibility', 'control' and 'getting on with things'.

In direct discussion on responsibility, all the men indicated that, although the health service had a duty to provide information regarding health issues, it was up to the individual to choose to act, or not, on this information and more will be said about this in Chapter 5. There were strong narratives about the need to take individual responsibility for health in terms of lifestyle choices. This contrasts markedly with views expressed in the health professional literature, and echoed here by the health professionals, which suggests, either overtly or covertly, that men fail to take matters relating to their health seriously and are irresponsible when it comes to caring for their health. This irresponsibility is usually implied through the use of phrases such as 'ignoring', 'complacent', 'neglectful' and that men are 'unaware' or see health as 'irrelevant' (for example, Fareed 1994; Griffiths 1999; Banks 2001). Yet, when giving direct examples of when and how they took responsibility for their health, all the men felt they had to provide some explanation for doing so; they could not be seen to be 'doing' health for its own sake. Not to provide an explanation would seem to run the risk of not being a (real) man and explanations were used to legitimate an interest in health thus allowing resolution of the 'don't care/should care' dichotomy.

This situation was slightly different for the gay men. The gay men themselves and the health professionals believed that gay men care more about their health than straight men (although this wasn't necessarily demonstrated in terms of actual health practices). It seems that the rise of HIV/AIDS, and the association of gay men with femininity, combined to legitimate, and perhaps even make a moral requirement, caring about health issues for gay men. This allowed them to dispense with a 'don't care' approach and was apparent in all the interviews with gay men and is summed up well by Gary: 'I think gay men are more aware of their health than straight men. I'm not saying that about all gay men and all straight men, but on the whole I think that gay men are more health conscious' (Gary, GM3).

However, this situating, or being situated, outside of hegemonic ideals, while legitimating individual concern with health, also situates gay men as 'other' in respect to hegemonic masculinity and thereby creates the stigma (and its concomitant impact on well-being) associated with homophobia and the material practices that serve to subordinate gay men mentioned earlier. It may also mean that gay men are under a greater imperative to be seen to care for their health and well-being and are therefore judged more harshly, including by their peers, should this appear not to be the case.

The moral role of individual responsibility for health also raises particular issues for those with chronic illness or physical impairment who, as Williams (1993) and Galvin (2002) suggest, may feel under more obligation to present themselves as virtuous.

Physical impairment or underlying pathology could therefore represent a further legitimate explanation for being concerned about health, a way of resolving the 'don't care/should care' dichotomy. Peter provides an example: 'I think, since I've been in the chair, I've watched what I've eaten because I can't lose it, cause I've got no sensation. I'm worried honestly about getting a belly and not being able to get rid of it cause I can't work it' (Peter, DM1).

In this sense, particular physical circumstances, for Peter being a wheel-chair user, can almost obliterate the 'don't care/should care' dichotomy, leaving a 'must care' model, again creating a greater imperative to make 'correct' lifestyle choices. Yet this risks being emasculating, moving these men towards the boundary between hegemonic masculine identity and a feminized, and thereby marginalized, identity. Losing the 'edge' represented by this dichotomy risks the loss of (hegemonic) masculine identity and some of these men specifically (re)inserted aspects of 'don't care' into their narratives, symbolically using the very 'vulnerability' that is meant to make them take (more) care, as a way of presenting who they are. As Quinn explains during a discussion on whether he wants to live a long life:

> I just don't think about it, never think about it. Like I'll go down the kerb right, most people in a wheelchair will turn round and go down backwards. I don't, I just go straight down the kerb you know, throw meself off it. [...] I mean if I fell out of the chair and hurt meself then, the way I think is just like able-bodied people, they just don't think about it and neither do I. If I get hurt, I get hurt. I've always been like that, I've always just got on with it.
>
> (Quinn, DM2)

Quinn is not trying to deny his impairment here, or the effects of it, but he is showing that his attitude or approach to life is the same as that of an 'able-bodied' person. Yet this person is not asexual. In drawing on the rhetoric of risk, danger and lack of concern, as well as suggesting his skill and control in the handling of his wheelchair, Quinn is expressly demonstrating his normal *male* attitude and approach to life. His 'not thinking about it' also reaffirms Bourdieu's (1990) point that such actions (including the way that they are gendered) are often unconsciously entered into, representing part of a 'practical logic' demonstrated in everyday life.

Yet, it is not just caring too much about health that puts hegemonic identity at risk. Not to take enough care with one's health, particularly through indulging in excess, also moves one away from hegemonic ideals. It suggests irresponsibility and lack of control, which then become representative of transgressive (male) behaviour, as the following conversation suggests:

> *Frank:* If you enjoy a burger, eat it. If there was a salad I didn't enjoy, and a burger that I would enjoy that was gonna do me more harm, I'm sorry but I'd eat the burger.
>
> *SR:* So part of living a full life is....
>
> *Frank:* Enjoy your life, yeah. *I think you have to be a bit sensible, you can't be totally brash, you have to be sensible and responsible to a point. There's a point and once you get past that point you're being silly again.* Some people are too careful; that's not me.
>
> *SR:* So it's a balance?
>
> *Frank:* Yeah, you've got to get it right, yeah.
>
> (Frank, DM6, emphasis added)

This narrative provides a strong sense of the work required in balancing not only the 'don't care/should care' dichotomy but also balancing the tension between control and release in order to achieve or maintain 'healthy' hegemonic, male citizenship.

Taking care or just good luck?

One area not yet covered in this chapter, but significant in some of the men's interviews, was the issue of fate and/or genetic predisposition with regard to health. For Tony (DM5), even though he had obvious and self-declared ongoing health problems, leaving him prone to chest infections, it was important for him to make clear to me that he had 'good resistance' for warding off possible infections. This presentation of health in the face of illness or impairment has previously been noted in Cornwell's (1984: 124*ff*) work and she suggests it serves the purpose of separating off the illness from individual responsibility or 'fault'. In addition though, given that current constructions of hegemonic masculinity revolve around notions of strength, or at least not admitting weakness, the rhetoric also serves the purpose of allowing the men to present themselves as essentially male; naturally strong and resilient. It is no surprise, then, that several of the men declared a pre-disposition towards good health with phrases such as 'I've always been healthy' or 'I don't seem to pick up illnesses' being relatively commonplace.

It was difficult to be clear whether notions about fate and luck were mobilized as a resistance to current thinking that individual lifestyle choices are responsible for health outcomes or whether they were being used by the men to legitimate what they perceived as 'unhealthy' lifestyle choices. They often seemed to involve elements of both:

> You could not drink, not eat unhealthily, do a lot of exercise and still you could end up in your 60s, 70s having a heart attack, a stroke or whatever. I think as long as you're not really, really pushing it to the limit all the time, I think if you're in moderation, you just have to take your lot, and take what comes.
>
> (Owen, CABS5)

The men seemed to use the element that chance played in the possible outcomes to explain situations when the duty to choose healthy lifestyles had not been adhered to. This was particularly noticeable in justifications of smoking. For some health professionals such rhetoric was seen *only* as an excuse for not wanting to change particular health practices:

> Smoking, alcohol or whatever, over those healthy limits they are taking a risk. But that kind of person will probably say 'Well I'm taking a risk when I cross the road, I might get knocked over by a bus.' That will probably be their attitude won't it? Cause they just don't think it will happen to them, do they?
>
> (Eve, HP6)

Although this was the main way that such rhetoric was mobilized, it sometimes seemed to represent something more. For Hugh, the use of rhetoric about luck or chance in relation to mortality seemed to provide a way to rationalize and survive some very distressing events, including death and bloodshed, he had witnessed during his time in the army. This puts issues about lifestyle choices into a different perspective for him:

> It's like I've always thought if your number's up, your number's up, no matter what you do. I could walk out and get knocked over. I've

> seen people in the army, these guys are 19, 20 years old, they don't
> drink, they don't smoke and they were dead before they were 24.
>
> (Hugh, CABS2)

In this sense, ideas about health outcomes as being a matter of luck or fate may be psychodiscursive practices mobilized to help people through difficult material circumstances and a mechanism for allowing the separation of illness, impairment and death from individual blame. The number of men here is only small, but it was noticeable that these fatalistic notions were most commonly used by the men from lower socio-economic backgrounds. This links in with Donovan's (1986) and Howlett et al.'s (1992) research suggesting that groups with least power in society are more likely to hold fatalistic views on health and illness causation. For working-class men particularly, as Connell (2000: 187*ff*) points out, their position in the labour market makes them particularly likely to have encountered, even if not directly, injury and increased mortality as a result of working practices or conditions. As with Hugh's experience in the army, taking a fatalistic view regarding health outcomes may provide a means of reconciling these encounters with continued engagement in such an environment for men.

This has implications for health promotion. As Davison et al. (1992) point out, claims about the effects of lifestyle choices based on predictability, regularity and aggregated data do not fit with such fatalistic lay beliefs and this was born out in discussions with the men that utilised these notions:

> Me Grandma, she's 90 year old, smoked all her life and there's nothing wrong with her [...] There's no proof that shows to me that smoking will kill you, it may help, but its like I still think if my time's up, me time's up, there's nothing you can do about it.
>
> (Hugh, CABS2)

A framework for understanding hegemonic masculinity and health

It is clear that the moral nature of health talk means that it is inevitably tied up with narratives of responsibility, risk and the requirements of 'good' citizenship. However, these narratives themselves are far from devoid of gendered context and the requirements for 'good' male citizenship can sometimes collide with, and at other times facilitate, what currently constitutes 'good' health practices.

A model emerges then (Figure 2.1) that signifies this relationship between the 'don't care/should care' dichotomy and issues of control and release and how they are mobilized in regard to the construction of hegemonic masculinity.

Just as masculinities are not static but rather represent configurations of gender practice that men move within and between, so the four elements

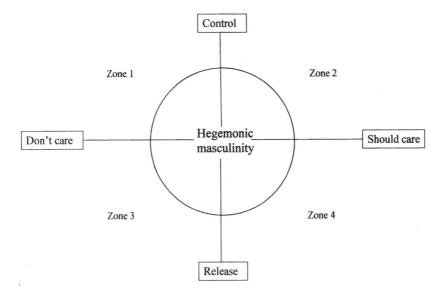

Figure 2.1

outlined in the model are mobilized in different ways at different times in order to achieve (or reject) hegemonic ideals. They are also contingent on other aspects of identity management, particularly the role that responsibility plays through the lifecourse. The holding together, or management, of these four aspects requires effort, although, as suggested previously, it is often achieved unconsciously as part of everyday life. Lack of ability, or desire, to hold these together can situate men in the four outer zones, that come to represent a symbolic 'no man's land'. This may be a deliberate positioning for some men, providing a place or space to challenge hegemonic ideals, but others are involved in an almost constant self-monitoring process, ensuring that they do not stray outside the 'inner circle' or 'target' that is hegemonic masculinity.

The men's accounts suggest that balance between 'healthy' control and release in relation to displaying hegemonic ideals may vary through the lifecourse. Younger or single men are expected to demonstrate some propensity towards excess (while not losing all control) and men in partnerships, particularly with children, are expected to demonstrate more control (whilst maintaining an air of 'dangerousness'). I suggest, after Wetherell and Edley (1999), that this might be because hegemonic ideals vary and are dependant on particular social sites. They suggest that focusing on hegemonic masculinity as a mode of self-presentation is too narrow as most situations require attention to multiple identity positioning. They reject Connell's (1995) model of gender/masculinity hierarchies in these terms, suggesting that his 'account of the discursive/ideological field is too neat' (Wetherell and Edley

1999: 352). However, I would argue that they misinterpret or misunderstand the notion of hegemony, which, for Connell, represents not only a powerful identity discourse that men draw on (or reject) in social interactions, but a pre-existing set of structural relations that also affects access to a range of material resources. As such, hegemony is only one of a plethora of narrative scripts that men can draw on (or reject) *but will always be structurally situated in respect of.* Thus for the gay men situating, or being situated, as caring about their health may be a requirement for demonstrating virtuous behaviour in a time of 'risk' from HIV/AIDS but that also, as outlined earlier, subordinates them in respect of hegemonic masculinity and thereby leaves them vulnerable to the personal and material effects of homophobia.

Lupton (1993) points out that 'risk' in recent times has become synonymous with danger and risk avoidance becomes a medium through which correct moral behaviour is recommended. As such, notions of risk in relation to health, she suggests, serve a social and political function. Yet, in applying this idea to men as healthy citizens, Petersen and Lupton (1996: 80*ff*) suggest a somewhat simplistic model where the taking of 'risks' becomes solely a vehicle that men use to demonstrate hegemonic masculinity. Accounts here suggest that whereas this model concurs with the beliefs of the health professionals interviewed, it oversimplifies the lived reality of the men themselves. There is a complex interplay between control and release, on one hand, and the morality attached to caring or not caring for one's health, on the other. *Both taking risks and the controlling of risks are vehicles used by the men, in different ways and at different times, in the formation and/or expression of hegemonic and other masculine identities.* This suggests that whereas what constitute 'risks' are, as Petersen and Lupton (1996) point out, socially constructed, these constructions are then used, mobilized and interpreted in a variety of ways, or rejected, in aspects of identity management.

Summary

It is clear that men conceptualized health in a variety of ways, generally in line with previous work on lay perceptions of health. Particular attention has been drawn to the importance for men of showing (at least publicly) indifference to health and that this is the primary way that men's attitude towards health was viewed by the health professionals. Yet this conflicts in late modernity with a drive towards 'healthism' (Crawford 1980), where the individual is expected to combine aspects of control and release in order to achieve and maintain a healthy lifestyle as a moral imperative. This 'healthy balance', and how it could and should be achieved, therefore also needs to be negotiated with regard to one's gendered identity. In this way, as Saltonstall (1993) suggests, 'doing' (and I would suggest giving the appearance of not doing) health therefore becomes a way of 'doing' gender.

The converse can also been seen to hold true from the data presented here; that is that 'doing' gender can be a way of 'doing' health. The requirement for control and release is also a requirement for demonstrating hegemonic masculinity and health can therefore become an arena, or medium, through which hegemonic values can be displayed. It is not just that health is thought about in terms of self-control but, as Crawford (1984: 77) points out, self-control as a Western value is thought about through health. To show self-control, particularly as part of male identity, is to be a responsible citizen and this control can be demonstrated through health practices. There is therefore a reciprocal and socially integrated relationship between 'health' and 'gender'.

The idea that men are irresponsible in health matters, rhetoric found in interviews with the health professionals and echoed in health professional journals, could be, at least partially, responsible for constructing this as a reality. Certainly narratives about 'macho', irresponsible behaviour were present in the interviews with men themselves although they mainly distanced themselves from currently engaging in such behaviour, usually using the homogenous terms 'men' rather than 'I', 'they' rather than 'we', in these narratives. The men also gave numerous accounts of times when they had taken responsibility for their health although they seemed to feel obliged to provide explanations as to why they had done so.

This chapter has concentrated primarily on the role that discourses of health and masculinity play in the formation of identity for men. However, this can give the appearance of the men as being disembodied, claiming identities only in relation to a range of available discourses. The following chapter takes these discussions forward by looking more closely at the embodied nature of the relationship between masculinity and health and the role that the body plays in such identity formation.

Key points

- Men's apparent non-consideration of 'health' reflects a wider public discourse that men are not, or should not be, interested in their health.
- Good citizenship requires caring for health thus creating a 'don't care/should care' dichotomy for men.
- Men linked feeling 'healthy' to 'functionality' and sets of life circumstances rather than the state of the physical body.
- Some groups of men, gay men and disabled, are under a greater moral imperative to be seen to care for their health and well-being.
- In the context of men's health, 'risk' is not about probability, or chance, of an event happening but is interwoven with maintaining an integral (hegemonic) male identity.

- The taking of 'risks' is often seen by men as a measured activity not as a reckless abdication of responsibility.
- Hegemonic masculine ideals alter across the lifecourse often shifting from 'taking risks' when young to 'controlling excess' when entering stable relationships and fatherhood.

Key points for practice

- The 'don't care/should care' dichotomy that men face in conceptualizing health creates opportunities for health practitioners who can help move men toward the 'should care' element.
- That 'feeling healthy' for men is about life circumstances suggests that health practitioners need to focus on understanding such circumstances and seeing where opportunities for change may have good fit rather than just focusing on the physical body or on altering 'behaviour'.
- Likewise, 'risks' in relation to men and health are not about individual men and their 'behaviour' but are about managing sets of power relations. Sustaining a hegemonic male identity requires both the taking of risks but also the ability to exert self-control and take responsibility. The balance between these often alters over men's lifecourse and again provides opportunity for promoting particular lifestyle choices.
- Health professionals can help men manage the 'don't care/should care' dichotomy by recognizing and providing the 'legitimation' men need to utilize health services.

Notes

1. Mullen (1993) and Watson (2000) suggest that health is defined by fitness for men and Blaxter (1990) and Saltonstall (1993), in comparing men's and women's lay perceptions, suggest that such a way of defining health is more common for men.
2. In Blaxter's (1990) work similar ideas are covered, or fall between, the concept of 'psycho-social well-being' and 'health as energy'. In Watson's (2000) work they are covered by the concept of 'health as well-being' and in Mullen's (1993) work under 'health as correct mental attitude'. Perhaps the lack of desire to directly understand 'health as feeling' stems from a more general reluctance to engage with the emotions in sociological work more generally as S.J. Williams (2001) has noted.
3. This is not to say other empirical research data would not support such a model. Indeed, work by Crossley (2002) suggests that the very identification

of an action being deemed 'risky' by health promotion experts may create the opportunity for transgressive activity; in the case of her research 'bare-backing', the deliberate non-use of condoms amongst gay men, exemplifies this.

4. Crawford (1984: 94*ff*) does not maintain that release or transgression cannot be a subversive activity, merely that it should not always be interpreted in this way, just as self-control cannot always be interpreted as acquiescing to dominant discourses but may itself represent a subversive act as in cases of extreme bodily discipline such as anorexia.

3   Embodied masculinities and health

Introduction

Having set the context and considered how the men conceptualized health, it is important to understand how these notions are influenced by, and have influence on, male bodies; that is, it is important to begin to explore how these conceptualizations are not merely abstract but become embodied in gendered interactions.

Theoretical work has uncovered a range of complexities and contradictions that often exist in the relationship between men and their bodies. Seidler (1994, 1997), for example, concentrates on how men have become disembodied within postenlightenment thinking and particularly the role of 'Cartesian dualism' (the way that mind and body became philosophically separated) in this process. He explores how this Cartesian 'mind/body' split had historical impact with men becoming associated with the mind and reason, and women with the body and nature. In this sense, women are postulated as more embodied and, conversely, men are said to have lost touch with their ability to listen to and understand their bodies. This view is certainly echoed in health professional literature where men are frequently postulated as having a 'mechanistic' view of their bodies (for example, Lloyd 2001; White 2001).

Yet, other work, such as Connell's (1995: 45), suggests that masculinity is inherently tied up within the issue of bodies and that 'true masculinity is almost always thought to proceed from men's bodies'. He suggests that the body therefore plays a key role in maintaining (often inequitable) gender relations, both those between men and women but also those between different groups of men. Still more recent theoretical work, linked to post-structuralist and postmodern feminist insights, has suggested that bodies, including male bodies, are 'discursively fabricated' in the process of exercising power/knowledge. White, European, middle-class, heterosexual male bodies become socially constructed as the 'norm' or standard by which other bodies are measured, becoming represented as 'other' and less worthy (Petersen 1998: 41*ff*).

The body has thereby become theoretically politicized and this leads to a situation where what constitutes the body, whether physical or social, material or cultural, experiential or representational, has become hotly contested (Williams 1999: 798).

Whilst such theoretical work is important, it is rarely grounded through empirical studies. The above literature has begun to explore aspects of embodied masculinity (see also Connell 1987; Morgan 1993) but only a small literature exists that explores how this may impact on health (Sabo and Gordon 1995; Buchbinder 1998; Connell 2000) and even fewer works provide empirical data that link embodied masculinity and health (Cameron and Bernardes 1998; Watson 2000; C. Williams 2000).

Sociology, particularly the sociology of health and illness, has historically treated the body implicitly rather than explicitly (Morgan and Scott 1993). This has changed significantly in recent years (Williams and Bendelow 1998a) but there has still been some reluctance to engage in sociological research focused on the body and therefore also empirical work on gendered embodiment. As Nettleton and Watson (1998: 2) point out:

> Given the centrality of the body to everyday life [...] it is perhaps surprising that there has been so little empirical investigation into the body. In particular, there has been little research which involves engaging ordinary men and women in talk about their bodily experiences.

The purpose of this chapter is to extend the available empirical research on gender, masculinity, embodiment and health. It takes as a starting point Turner's (1992: 57) premise that the body should be regarded as 'simultaneously both discursive and animated, both *Körper* and *Leib*, both socially constructed and objective'. With this in mind, the first section concentrates on demonstrating the reality of the physical body, and its relation to gender, health and well-being, through men's accounts of everyday experiences. Having done this, the second section then explores the importance of bodily representations, and particularly normative gendered bodily representations, in relation to health and well-being. The third section then considers how male bodies move through place and space and the relationship of this to health practices.

Experiencing the body

This section begins to develop, through lay men's own accounts, the how, when and where of the real physical body in respect to health and well-being. In Chapter 1 I introduced Watson's (2000: 115*ff*) 'male body schema' as a way to understand how embodiment can be seen as existing in four interrelated ways in respect to men, health and well-being. The schema, presented again below, is used in this section as a framework for progressing Watson's work by further exploration of physiological (visceral) embodiment and its relationship to experiential and pragmatic embodiment and health practices.

The notion of normative embodiment will be explored later in the chapter as it relates more directly to issues of appearance and body image.

Table 3.1 Watson's (2000) 'male body schema'

Normative embodiment	'Normal', 'standard' or idealized accounts of bodily shape(s).
Pragmatic embodiment	The functional use of a 'normal everyday body' in order to fulfil specific roles ('father', 'husband', 'worker') required in the social world.
Experiential embodiment	The point of contact of social and physical boundaries, the primary site for experience of emotion and physicality.
Visceral embodiment	The indirect biological processes, usually unconsciously experienced, that support bodily function and, to an extent, determine bodily shape.

Everyday bodies

All the health professionals interviewed saw physical, bodily activity, usually termed 'exercise' and seen as a discrete area of activity, as being a significant contributor to health and well-being. This seemed to be primarily and very specifically related to the continued and correct functioning of an inner, physical body. This view was also articulated by some of the men interviewed, as Bob explains:

> I enjoy an active lifestyle. I go out sometimes just for a walk, that to me, contributes to your health. If you exercise, your body is a mass of muscle, if you exercise your muscle it'll last longer, it has better tone and works better. My hobbies are all active, I mean kite buggying is very strenuous, and gym, I enjoy the gym as well. The fitness side of things is a big contributory factor to your health.
>
> (Bob, CABS6)

Yet, it is clearly far more than just the working of the inner body that was of significance to the men and, as Bob's remarks suggest, bodily activity is socially integrated; it is related as much, if not more, to experiential embodiment as it is to physiological processes. It is clear that, for most of the men, what it is to be healthy is a corporeal experience realized in and through everyday activities. Thus, when defining health, it is Owen's body *as experienced in everyday life* that signifies to him whether a new 'health' regime (dietary changes and increase in exercise) is having an effect:

It's feeling good when you wake up in the morning, that's one of the things I've found since things have changed, just not feeling lack-adaisical. Being able to walk a few flights of stairs and not puffing and panting. I find I sleep better at night since things have changed over the last month. I just seem more alert really, a lot healthier. I'm not there yet, but I feel a lot healthier which helps at work and at home and everything else [. . .] The breathing's important, I think that's the main thing you notice when you're a bit out of shape. I always used to get the lift at work, three flights of stairs, but now I don't, I walk and it's getting easier and easier. You can tell when you get to the top, sit at your desk and two minutes later you can talk again sort of thing.

(Owen, CABS5)

This is representative of what Watson (2000: 118) terms 'pragmatic embodiment', the most common level of embodiment presented by the men in his study. Pragmatic embodiment, he suggests, is about the functional use of a 'normal everyday body' in order to fulfil specific, and often multiple, roles ('father', 'husband', 'worker') required in the social world. Watson (2000: 136) considers how, by concentrating on underlying physical processes (what he terms the 'visceral body', accessed indirectly through taking a medical history and examination), health professionals at a well-man clinic often failed to explore individual men's pragmatic mode of embodiment. In not exploring this, there was a concomitant failure to recognize how health practices are rarely central to men's lives but are usually contingent upon, and secondary to, other aspects of their daily life. The accounts here support Watson's view that health professionals and men often, though not always, conceptualize the (male) body and its relation to health and health practices differently and that this has implications regarding access to, and the effectiveness of, health promotion initiatives. This is explored in more detail in Chapter 5.

Watson (2000: 119) further suggests that pragmatic embodiment leads to the 'losing', or marginalization, of the body for men. In arguments that reflect Parsons' (Parsons and Bales 1956) work on instrumental (male) roles and expressive (female) roles, he suggests that, as a tool or instrument used to fulfil gendered social roles, particularly physical labour, the male body becomes objectified and lost as the 'primary mode for experiencing the social world'. Similar arguments are made by Seidler (1989: 64) who states that, as men, 'We have little on-going relationship with our somatic processes. The body is to be used as an instrument to serve ends, rather than to be listened to'. Yet, whilst these men's narratives did represent the body as a tool or instrument for fulfilling gendered social roles, this was not the sole or even primary narrative and the materiality of physical bodies also acted as the touchpoint of subjective engagement with the social world:

Say like me, your job, you're sat at your desk all day, you're basically bored, just doing your job, going home, and that's [sport] your release. You know, you're getting out there letting all, not so much the frustrations, but you've got all this pent-up energy inside you in a way and you've got to get rid of it [. . .] That's what I said to them in Badminton last week, I said, 'I've been like a coiled spring this last week', I just wanted to get out and do something.

(Francis, CABS1)

Francis' boredom with work is felt by and in his body, it is embodied, and the solution is therefore also found in release through the experiential body; through the subjective experiences of physical engagement in the world. This is not to deny the importance of understanding the implications of pragmatic embodiment. Both the source of Francis' boredom and the choice of release are related to aspects of his gendered pragmatic embodiment. As Bourdieu (1979: 191*ff*) outlines, bodies become shaped through these daily, unconscious, practices that are socially located and gender specific. Thus he points out that 'it behoves a man to eat and drink more, and to eat and drink stronger things' and this with 'whole-hearted male gulps and mouthfuls'. What I am suggesting is that these gendered forms of embodiment *are* experienced subjectively, as experiential embodiment, as well as pragmatically, by the men and that they are recognized as being effected through, and having an effect on, a real physical, visceral body. As Watson (2000: 139*ff*) suggests, pragmatic male embodiment should therefore form a significant area of interest for those wishing to improve the health of men. Biological and individual behavioural explanations regarding men and health, proffered by the health professionals interviewed, often failed to recognize the significance of pragmatic embodiment to health practices and outcomes and its relationship, through experiential embodiment, to physiological processes.

Invisible physicality?

Whilst to an extent taken for granted and hidden in everyday life, the existence of a real, physical body, and its relation to health and well-being, was still significant for the men, being confirmed for them through felt bodily experiences; that is, through experiential embodiment. Examples of this were provided by what Monaghan (2001) terms 'vibrant physicality', the embodiment of feeling healthy or well: 'I started getting into me fitness and four years ago, when I tried basketball, fell in love with it [. . .] Totally fell in love with it, brilliant sport, came off, good sweat, heart pumping, adrenaline rushing, excellent, loved it.' (Peter, DM1).

Examples were more frequently found when experiential embodiment suggested that there was a problem with these hidden, physiological processes:

Originally, I had a weak ankle for about 14 months and I kept going every month to see Dr S. and he said 'Oh you've got psoriasis in your bone.' So I said 'I've never heard of psoriasis in the bone before.' 'Oh yeah' he said. So after about 14 months I just said to him 'I'm getting a bit sick of this now. I'm coming every month, I'm having this injection, I'm doing this, I'm strapped up, me boots, I'm even getting smaller boots to keep me ankle really tight and solid because I keep on going over on it, what are we gonna do about it?' So he says 'Well we'd better do a biopsy, but I won't be able to do it, I'll put you in touch with someone else.' So they put me in touch with someone else and did the biopsy and it was cancer. So I was a little bit, I were a little bit peed off really because I didn't wanna see Dr S. again cause I thought, well, he might have been able to save me foot 14 month ago.

(Vernon, DM4)

Changes in physiological processes (the spreading of cancer cells) affected Vernon's experiential embodiment (his ability to walk without 'going over' on his ankle) and interrupted his pragmatic embodiment (his ability to carry out his roles in daily life) leading him to seek help. Contrary to the health professionals' views that men have a singularly mechanical view of their bodies (often echoed in health professional literature – for example, Griffiths 1999; Lloyd 2001), the men in this study provided many unsolicited examples of learning through both their own and other's experiential embodiment:

I have the attacks so often, every 12 weeks I have a serious attack in either both legs or just one and that's the medication wearing off. So even though you learn to live with it, and you learn to live within your environment, and you try to act the tough person, doing this and doing that, some days you're just not able to do it.

(Ron, DM3)

I'd mention it [aching in hands] to my dad who would probably know better than them [GPs] to be honest. I'd ask me dad cause he's had experience of it [rheumatoid arthritis] for 15 years. He has injections regularly which keeps it under control, which means he can get on with his everyday life. It will get to a time where he can't which I'm sure he's got his head round cause he's known its coming a long time.

(Owen, CABS5)

In this sense experiential embodiment, a subjective knowing through the body, was seen as being important in both recognizing the emergence of changing physiological processes but also in knowing how to live with such changes, the adjustments that might need to be made to facilitate continued pragmatic embodiment.

The idea that these physiological processes were taken for granted also seems to imply that they are not consciously thought about unless they interrupted or punctured daily life, a view strongly expressed by most of the health professionals:

> People don't have concerns about health until it goes wrong [...] And if the body is something that works perfectly well then don't worry about it until it goes wrong, in much the same way as your car I suppose. People don't get their car serviced particularly frequently; they only get it done when it breaks down.
>
> (John, HP3)

Such narratives were certainly echoed by all the men interviewed. However, there was also awareness amongst the men that underlying physiological processes acted to support daily functioning; that is, physiological embodiment was a basis for pragmatic embodiment. At times these processes were presented in terms of a self-monitoring and self-regulating system: 'My outlook on it is, if there is anything wrong with me I leave it to the body to repair itself. I'm not one if I get the sniffles, I don't take tablets, I don't take medicines' (Hugh, CABS2).

Such an approach is not an abdication of responsibility and later in the interview, when discussing well-man clinics, Hugh goes on to explain:

> I'd go along. I mean there are certain things like I think to myself 'Is there something going on in my body that I don't know about?' And you'd find out then wouldn't you. It's like I say if there is something wrong with me I want to know as soon as possible so I can do something about it, I want to be given the best fighting chance to do something about it.
>
> (Hugh, CABS2)

Saltonstall (1993) has outlined how men seem to have a 'power-over' relationship with their bodies, yet Hugh's remarks suggest a situation more complex. Hugh's comments suggest that he would want to work (fight) *with* the (natural) physiological bodily processes rather than thinking he can control them. This takes a specific gendered form when discourses of discipline are inserted and such narratives are particularly present in the interviews with Hugh (as in the quote above) and Bob, both ex-army men:

> Since [going into hospital for MS] I've been relatively OK as long as you manage it properly. I gave up smoking, cut my alcohol intake

right down and gave up coffee. I've started to manage my food as well, cut out saturated fat completely to give my body a chance basically.

(Bob, CABS6)

The need for bodily discipline is a significant part of these men's (male) identities yet is contingent on specific circumstances. If alerted through experiential embodiment that physiological processes are 'faulty' *and not self-correcting*, then there is a moral obligation (see also Chapter 2) to provide the (natural, physical) body with the best chance of recovery. It is possible that it is this process that leads to the high levels of compliance with medical regimes found amongst some men in previous research on chronic illnesses (Gordon 1995; Cameron and Bernardes 1998; C. Williams 2000). Yet, as Charmaz (1995: 287) points out, this desire to preserve a public (male) identity based on disciplining the body can also be damaging in the long term, particularly if the desired identity cannot be sustained as physiological processes continue to deteriorate and no or few alternative narrative identities are provided to draw on.

Changing bodies

Physiological processes were also seen as variable and subject to change. This change could be due to having a 'natural', usually seen as hereditary, pre-disposition towards particular changes, or the 'natural' decline of the body with age, or a combination of these:

My dad's got rheumatoid arthritis. You know, my granny had it, my dad had it, so I'm always worried whether I'm gonna get it. If I ever get any aches and pains in me hands, or me wrists or fingers, I'm always thinking, 'Is this the start?'

(Owen, CABS5)

I think as I'm getting a bit older, I'm nearly 40, you get more aches and pains and things like that and you start thinking about things a bit more.

(Kiaran, GM4)

However, changes to physiological processes, including 'natural' chan-ges, were also seen, at least to some degree, to be dependent on aspects of experiential embodiment, particularly what goes into the body and the risks associated with excess. At times, the desire to pursue a 'healthy' experiential form of embodiment, vibrant physicality achieved through sport, drink, drugs, food, or (particularly for the gay men) sex, clashed with the anticipated effects of this on physiological processes. *The tension between control and release, discussed in the previous chapter, is in this sense played out at the interface between the physiological and experiential body:*

> *Dan:* Like most people now, especially men, you'll have a salad, you'll have a tuna sandwich, you'll eat a lot more healthily and be a lot more conscious of it [health]. But then you'll have a blow out, like last night, I'll go out and do what ever I want, smoke what I want, drink what I want, eat what I want. So it's a binge, look after yourself for five days a week in general and then hammer yourself for two.
>
> *SR:* And do you think that in itself can be quite healthy?
>
> *Dan:* I think it can be, mentally it gives you like a stress release factor [. . .] I think your body can generally adapt if it gets a regular intake of whatever you give it, but if you shock it every week I think it thinks 'Jesus, what's going on here?'
>
> (Dan, CABS7)

There was a sense, then, of responsibility towards the physiological body that had to be held in balance with the desire to pursue corporeal pleasure. This sense of responsibility, the need to 'help', care for, or be vigilant regarding the body, was particularly marked when chronic illness or physical impairment threatened either physiological or pragmatic embodiment:

> Because I'm disabled, I've got health problems as well, I keep as healthy as I can because I've also got asthma and I pick up bugs quite easily. The workers [carers] have got to be careful, if they've got a bad cold they can't come to work because I'll catch it and would be much iller than them. I've got quite good resistance but obviously we have to be careful because if I catch it, it'll take me a week to get over it and cause umpteen other problems.
>
> (Tony, DM5)

This need to have an element of vigilance regarding underlying physiological processes was, then, often contingent upon other aspects of identity – for Tony his increased susceptibility through physical impairment. For many of the gay men, such vigilance was centred on sexual health – no surprise given, as outlined in the previous chapter, how health is presented to and conceptualized by gay men:

> I mean we know a lot of people on the scene and off the scene. And a lot of people start out if there's something wrong they always say 'I've got this rash' or something like that, and the friends say, 'Oooooh I had a rash, I got some ointment from the chemist you

> know.' And of course there's a rash and there's a rash, there's two different things. So they might be doing something that at the end of the day, because they haven't gone straight to the people who can give advice and help them, they are putting their lives at risk you know or their future health at risk.
>
> (Wayne, GM6)

While recognizing that this vigilance is mediated through issues of identity, and is undoubtedly linked in part to morality and the need to appear virtuous (as discussed in the previous chapter), there are also issues about very real threats to bodily integrity, to physiological processes, further highlighted by Vernon:

> Eleven, 12 years later, you still live everyday as it comes. Sometimes when you feel a lump somewhere or summits not right you tend to think 'Shit, has it [cancer] come back?' Cause it was just gone five years after [the amputation] when I found I had a tumour round me nipple.
>
> (Vernon, DM4)

In concluding this section, the reality for Vernon of losing a leg, the subsequent loss of his breast, and similar narratives regarding physiological processes given by all the other men interviewed, suggest that the (male) body is not and cannot be seen *only* as a discursive fabrication. At the same time, a concentration by health professionals *only* on physiological processes, removed from men's experiential and particularly pragmatic embodiment, is unlikely to provide an adequate understanding of men's health practices in the context of their everyday lives. Physiological processes both affect and are affected by men's pragmatic embodiment and the experiential body acts as the site of recognition of this two-way process.

Bodily appearance and image

Having established a solid and tangible element to men's physicality, this section intends to explore the importance of cultural representations in respect of embodied masculinity and health. The argument in the previous section was not that men's bodies were not discursively constructed but that they were not *only* discursively constructed. The aim of this section, then, is to begin to show how cultural representations of embodied masculinity found in the men's accounts impact on health and well-being.

Looking good, feeling good

Previous work on lay perceptions of health has suggested that men are more inclined to think of health in terms of bodily function rather than appearance (Blaxter 1990: 24; Saltonstall 1993). Nevertheless, bodily shape and appearance, particularly as they related to a normative, desirable body, were clearly significant to these men with narratives about 'weight' and/or 'fat' being present in most of the interviews:

> Like I say I have problems with me weight, it fluctuates up and down so I feel healthier if I lose a bit of weight [...] When I was about 19 I went on a diet and lost about three stone which obviously helps, you feel a lot better cause you're getting more ... better looks from all the females of course, more self-confidence in a way.
>
> (Francis, CABS1)

For Francis, and several other men, the healthy aspects of being the 'correct' (normative) weight were as much related to benefits to the experiential body – 'if you look good, you feel good' – and the cultural capital that can accrue from this, as they were to benefits to physiological processes. Recent experiences of dieting (as above) were frequently used to signify a virtuous concern with health and being overweight was seen as a visual signifier of poor health (see also Watson 2000: 78). In this respect, women were postulated as being more concerned about their health (as appearance) than men by most of the men interviewed and by the health professionals. As Ian explains when considering why more women than men made use of an 'exercise on prescription' programme for depression:

> *Ian:*   I can't help thinking that the women's motivation was to lose weight. I would say that was more their priority rather than getting shot of the depression. Besides which, I think women are more committed to their health than men anyway, women tend to be more bothered and more likely to make the effort.
>
> *SR:*   Do you think that's related to what you were saying, to do with weight and image or is it to do with health directly?
>
> *Ian:*   I think its more to do with weight and the image, it kind of crosses a boundary, people I suppose are aware, if they are overweight the chances are they are not that healthy.
>
> (Ian, HP4)

As other studies have also suggested (Boroughs and Thompson 2002; Grogan and Richards 2002; Henwood et al. 2002), many of the men believed that male concern with bodily appearance was becoming more culturally acceptable and a few believed that working towards an ideal, normative body could help promote a positive, male, self-identity:

> About 10/12 years ago I lost something like three stone and your self-esteem grows, you look better, you feel better so your whole round persona improves. And a similar thing 3/4 years ago, I did a little sport, got myself a bit fitter, and felt better for doing it.
>
> (Francis, CABS1)

This was seen as a recent, historical change that was liberating yet also as having the potential to unhinge hegemonic male identity:

> That's the difference I see now with men. There's a surge in marketing which is ... The effect of that is beauty, vanity which has spread through from women to men. It's always been there but it's just not been talked about. Now it's full on and men are cashing in on it. It's the body beautiful effect, I mean it's always been for women you know, fat's in, thin's in, tall is in, small is in, and it's just maybe caught up with men. As in it's now known for a man to go out ... Not completely, obviously men hide it more. They've not got to the stage of putting make-up on and God help us if they did, well they do actually, what have I said! But not obviously in the general mainstream.
>
> (Dan, CABS7)

Shilling (1993: 3) suggests that in late modernity it is 'the exterior territories, or surfaces, of the body that symbolise the self'. The drive towards consumption (highlighted in Dan's quote above) is linked to the rise in the importance of the body as a project that can provide ontological security in terms of one's individual identity; the body becomes representative of who we are. In a time of uncertainty and risk one can retain at least a degree of control through working on the body-self; almost a literal moulding of oneself. As mentioned, this was the case for some of the men. Yet traditional cultural representations of hegemonic masculinity, that (real) men are unconcerned with bodily appearance this being the domain of women and gay men, also persisted for other men creating a tension in identity formation. Such tensions were sometimes resolved by the men through narratives that linked bodily appearance with specifically gendered activities, particularly sport and work. As Frank suggests when asked about a time when he had felt healthy or well:

> Particularly healthy? Well, when I was about 18 till about 21. I wouldn't say I was big, but I was certainly more muscular than I am

now, I had a six pack and everything. I used to work on [leisure park] as a maintenance guy, it keeps you fit, its heavy work and it builds your muscles up.

(Frank, DM6)

In this way, gendered discourses around health and the body can converge and the pragmatic body becomes instrumental in the development of a normative, healthy (male) body, achieved 'naturally' rather than by paying specific attention to it (see also Grogan and Richards 2002).

The strong action man

Current hegemonic masculinity continues to be constructed and maintained partly through the marginalization and subordination of women and non-heterosexual men (Connell 1995). It remains important therefore to identify 'difference' in order to sustain power relations, and the body, and how it is presented, is a key site for doing this. To an extent hegemonic masculine identity continues to be represented in embodied forms based on action and strength:

SR: So what are the things that keep you healthy do you think?

Quinn: Moving. Yeah cause a mate of mine he's in a wheelchair and ever since he's been a child he's not done anything and he's like a seven stone weakling basically. His wrists are about half the size of mine and he's really thin and his fingers are like witches, really thin fingers, and he can't walk. [...] All his life he's let people do it for him. If he wanted to go out he used to get hold of the back of my chair and I used to pull him from his house to town and back, it was an all day job [...] And I dare say I could be the same if I hadn't kept myself active.

(Quinn, DM2)

To be passive, to be thin and weak, is representative of an unhealthy, specifically male, body, suggestive as it is of stereotypical feminine characteristics, even being likened to a witch, something generally used to indicate that which is female, ugly and repugnant. Despite his own increasing physical impairment, Quinn can therefore use 'health' talk to demonstrate his male identity through bodily representation metaphorically juxtaposed to that which is feminine. This representation of masculinity in terms of action and strength can also be problematic if changes in physiological processes, impairment or chronic illness, make the presentation of such normative, male embodiment difficult to sustain (Robertson 2004). It can raise concerns about one's gendered identity:

SR: With all the changes then [becoming physically impaired], has that changed the way you think of yourself as a man?

Vernon: Yeah, cause you don't ... though you know you're still a man and I've ended up in a chair, I don't feel like a red blooded man, you know. I don't feel I can handle 10 pints and get a woman and just do the business with them and forget it, like most young people do. You feel compromised and still sort of feeling like 'Will I be able to satisfy my partner?' Not just sexually, other ways, like DIY, jobs round the house and all sorts.

The construction of masculine embodiment in terms of drinking, sexual prowess and skilled labour, means Vernon has to (re)consider his male identity when these can no longer be maintained. He goes on to describe how many of the concerns he highlights are those that naturally occur for all men as they go through the process of maturing, settling down, and experiencing 'natural' wear and tear of the physical body. In this sense, one's gendered (male) identity becomes mediated by health experiences, through experiential embodiment, and it is possible that disabled men could therefore provide role models for renegotiating masculine identity through such life-course transitions (Shakespeare 1999: 57).

Shakespeare (1994) outlines how, historically, disabled people, like women, have come to represent the 'other' with regard to normative bodies. More than this, though, he argues that, as a visual reminder to able-bodied people of their own potential vulnerability, disabled people also represent a threat to notions of bodily invincibility and this is intrinsically tied up with masculinity through concerns with potency, supremacy and domination. That disabled people are actively posited as 'other', as 'dustbins for disavowal', and that this has material consequences, is attested to in all the interviews with disabled men and was felt to have a negative impact on their health and well-being. For those disabled men in wheelchairs the commonest form that this took was literally being 'talked over': 'You do get bad experiences off the public when you're out in a chair and people will talk over my head to [wife] and they'll completely ignore me' (Quinn, DM2).

The presence of physical impairment was also often seen as implying mental impairment and led to the rendering of the men as non-people or invisible:

In a wheelchair, people look at you and think there's obviously something wrong with your head [...] I go into a shop with [wife], buy something, and they don't talk to me, they give the change to [wife] and it's not a myth, it still happens today.

(Peter, DM1)

Bodies are integral to these encounters. Yet the disabled men were far from passive victims. Rather, they were frequently active agents in resisting and challenging such prejudice (see also Reeve 2002) and this often took a specific, embodied, gendered form as Frank shows:

> People will close the door on you on purpose if they see you coming in the chair, I've seen them do it. And I'll say something if they do. [Other people] feel they have to shout cause I'm in a chair, I'm not deaf you know. If they did it once and I told them and they didn't do it again, fair enough. But if they kept on doing it that would annoy me and if they didn't know I could stand up then I'd stand up and tell them face to face. If they won't listen then I'll intimidate them so they will listen, cause it's important. In a way it's taking the Mickey by shouting at me.
>
> (Frank, DM6)

Frank draws (perhaps unconsciously) on normative embodied aspects of male imagery – tall, strong, and (potentially) violent – in order to challenge what he has first established as deliberate prejudice yet is also perceived as a threat to his male pride. Given the importance of such embodied encounters in the disabled men's narratives, it is clear that the micro-social management of these personal encounters (see also Goffman 1968, 1969) cannot be overlooked in preference to social models of disability that only consider issues of structure to be significant such that 'disablement has nothing to do with the body' (Oliver 1996: 42). Yet neither can such micro-social management be divorced from the social context in which it occurs and the ideological and material structures that can create or restrict particular possibilities for individuals. It is unlikely (though not impossible) that a woman could draw on such imagery, use her body in the same way as Frank, and achieve the same results; agency must be placed firmly in specific, pre-existing yet continually reproduced, historical systems of domination. Frank, through social meanings invested in his biological sex, has the opportunity to draw on gendered bodily representations in this encounter and in doing so also acts to reproduce the idea(l) of male strength and domination.

Body images

It is not merely the appearance of the body, therefore, that is of significance, but the way that adornment, gesture, and movement combine to present an image and the culturally constructed meanings inherent in such images. There was a strong feeling among many of the men, and the health professionals, that the process of presenting a particular 'macho' image (or its more recent (re)incarnation, 'laddism') to friends was integrally tied to particular, potentially detrimental, health practices:

> *SR:* One of the things that came out of the focus groups was whether men felt more obliged, pressured, to participate in activities that were seen as detrimental to health . . .
>
> *Fiona:* Like drinking and peer group pressure, yeah. It's difficult to separate whether it is peer group pressure or if they really want to do it isn't it? Certainly men have more risky lives don't they in terms of trauma, driving fast cars, smoking and drinking at work, they're with their peers a lot more than a mother with three children aren't they?
>
> (Fiona, HP7)

Research by Canaan (1996); Gough and Edwards (1998) and Capraro (2000) all provide detailed accounts of the processes by which masculine identities become integrated with such health practices.

Sometimes, what people (men) want to do and what they feel pressure to do are not necessarily separable in the way suggested. Social practices and bodily dispositions, the image one wishes to present, the manner in which individuals 'carry themselves', what Bourdieu (1990) terms 'bodily hexis', are often socially and unconsciously inscribed as Dan suggests:

> There's also a danger factor like I said. You do all this keep-fit, looking good, feeling good but there's this growing trend in drugs, alcohol, looking cool, as in need a cigarette to look it [. . .] You can keep generally fit, but smoking, drugs and drink are a massive factor. And they do go hand in hand with looking good and getting the image.
>
> (Dan, CABS7)

In this sense, construction and maintenance of 'images' carries with it implied practices that impact on health and well-being. Yet such inscription is not deterministic and bodily deportment is at least partly contingent on specific social circumstances and subject to change. For the gay men, 'camping it up' represented such a specific combination, of adornment, gesture and movement, being representative of a shared identity and signifying one as part of the 'gay community'. This was often done in deliberate and specific contrast to (hegemonic) male images based on aggression and domination:

> If you're out with mates you're this butch man who's out with their butch mates and have got to be in charge, pick a fight and shout down the street at women because it's a manly thing to do [. . .] We're [gay men] more camping it down the street, shouting out to guys,

being a bit more camp and outrageous about things. Probably a bit more down to earth, cause we're havin' a laugh more than a big marching, you know, army march down the road. So it's probably the total opposite to traditional straight men.

(David, GM1)

Yet, as Linneman (2000) also points out, the risks involved meant that care and control had to be exercised over the when and where of such presentation: 'When I go out drinking and I go to a gay bar and I'm amongst friends I do sometimes camp it up a little bit, which I certainly wouldn't dream of doing normally. But in that sort of environment I do' (Gary, GM3).

A lot of gay people feel intimidated getting a crowd together say to go bowling or something like that cause they'd probably get a load of hassle. I mean everybody should be allowed to do what they like but if you get somebody [male] that's 27 stone in a pair of stiletto's and a miniskirt walking up [rough area of town] at 2 in the morning, you're really asking for it. You have to be sensible I think.

(Edward, GM2)

In this respect, whilst certain bodily dispositions may be culturally inscribed, this does not negate the role of agency in bodily deportment and presentation of self, particularly when specific images are required for the development of cultural capital and/or for reasons of personal protection.

Interacting elements

It is clear then that all four elements of the 'male body schema' continually interact, not only with each other but also with the men's conceptualizations of health, to influence health practices but also wider social interactions that impact on health and well-being.

This process of interaction, and its outcomes, are often mediated through issues of identity. In this way identity becomes the pivotal point of contact between the material and the representational as Moss and Dyke (1996: 474) suggest: 'Coming to terms with the disjuncture between one's own body and its representations is important in defining the boundaries of individual identities: boundaries that are continually adjusting.'

Whilst this statement was made in respect to chronic illness, as others have pointed out (McDowell 1999: 61), it remains just as applicable to the 'well' body. Whilst the representation of normative male body imagery was seen as desirable and 'healthy' to some, it was also frequently seen as a powerful factor in the production of particularly negative health practices, particularly drinking, smoking, fighting and risk taking.

Such normative representations were frequently subverted or resisted, but also utilized, when circumstances required it. For example, the gay men moved into and out of 'camp' (and 'straight') presentations of masculinity depending on the risks and advantages felt to be involved. Likewise, the disabled men developed a variety of strategies that relied on, reformulated, and rejected hegemonic masculinity (see also Gerschick and Miller 1995) to come to terms with (re)presenting what constituted male embodiment.

Yet, as others (Forrest 1994) have shown, the opportunity to 'choose' identities in this way is not equally open to all; as Warde (1992: 26) puts it 'people play with the signs they can afford'. Dominant social structures, particularly here heterosexism and disablism (integral components of current hegemonic masculinity), act to limit the role that agency could play at times in subverting, resisting or using hegemonic masculine imagery. Normative male bodily representations are built into structures as means of supporting or maintaining dominant systems, often by restricting physical access to material resources.

In concluding this section, it seems clear that bodies can be viewed as both objects and agents of practice (Connell 1995: 61). The men were at various times subject to socially prescribed normative (male) bodily representations. The pursuit of such an idealized, normative body provided feelings of achievement and positive identity for some men. However, the presentation of desirable, idealized male imagery in consumer culture was also seen as being linked to representations of 'machoism' or 'laddism' that incorporated negative health practices particularly drinking, fighting, smoking and drug taking, and was also damaging when such imagery could not be maintained. Such imagery was certainly not unquestioningly embraced by the men who were often active agents in the use, and specific non-use, of such normative representations; bending them, rejecting them or working around them to maximize their own advantage.

Bodies in place and space

The process of (male) identity formation, then, is clearly not just something achieved by individuals in isolation; it is not simply intrapsychic, occurring and being sustained within the confines of one's own mind. Rather it is intersubjective, formed and re-formed through interactions in everyday life, through the movement of real bodies in real space, yet also influenced by normative bodily representations. The aim of this section is to bring together the ideas presented so far in the preceding two sections of this chapter to explore further how the material and cultural, experiential and representational aspects of (male) embodiment combine and interface with health and well-being.

Locating bodies

It was clear that growing up in areas that provided sufficient, safe and pleasant space to play was important for some of the men interviewed:

> *SR:* Do you think your health is affected by where you live?
>
> *Martin:* It can only have a positive effect. When we were kids we used to do nothing but run around on the green all evening, all day, as soon as we finished school, at weekends. Certainly I think if you lived in a big city where there isn't such a large expanse of sort of grass area, I think … I've been fit all me life because of it really. And you can run the streets even after dark and again it keeps you fit, it keeps you active, whereas in large cities always 'got to be in by half seven'. So I think certainly living in such a nice area, a safe area it contributes directly to your health. There's clean air, it's not like living in London where, if you play sport in London, you're breathing in all the crap.
>
> (Martin, CABS3)

For Martin, the environment contributes indirectly to health through experiential embodiment, feelings of enjoyment through play and feeling safe, but also directly to physiological embodiment, keeping underlying processes robust and free from potentially harmful pollutants. Four of the health professionals also made clear links between men's immediate environment and the effect on health. For example, when discussing the mental health needs of men in his (deprived) practice area John, a GP, states:

> I think there is a fine line between constitutional unhappiness and actual depression [...] It's really sorting out social circumstances that would be good. So for instance, try to get all the bed-sit accommodation improved and improve B&B accommodation. Improve opportunities for non-skilled work to be available and make that more acceptably paid.
>
> (John, HP3)

There is a contrast here to much of health professionals' concentration on men's physiological embodiment and the effects of men's individual behaviour (narratives about excessive drinking, smoking and risk taking) on this. John offers insight into how improvements in men's pragmatic embodiment (housing, work) could improve experiential embodiment by raising self-esteem. In this way healthy (male) bodies are seen to be as much the product of healthy public policies as they are of individual behaviour(s). Yet, the 'healthy' male citizen continues to be one constructed through gender stereotypes, in this case the active breadwinner, and this is discussed further shortly.

Environment and health practices were also linked through representations of culturally specific normative embodiment, as Ian suggests: 'The trouble with [town] is it's a very pub-orientated market town, still a very 'macho' image, and there's a big alcohol culture. There's also a huge drugs culture with the younger men, huge by all accounts' (Ian, HP4).

Through such representations, particular public places become marked out as gendered spaces. Whilst such spaces are not the sole province of men and male bodies, those who enter them are certainly subject to informal, hegemonic masculine rules governing appropriate embodied behaviour (Hey 1986; McDowell 1999) and this is seen to have implications for health and well-being; required behaviours may be destructive to physiological processes. That hegemonic masculinity is constructed through heterosexuality also leads to the marginalization of other groups from these gendered spaces. The care that the gay men had to take in bodily deportment in public places and spaces, outlined at the end of the previous section, led to the carving out of specific and safe public spaces:

> Gay men tend to socialize a lot because they're all stuck together in one, well not many, places. I think we're closer because of the prejudice against gay people, so we've got our own little clubs. And somewhere like [town] I think there's what four, five clubs [...] Yeah, cause that's the only place that gay men really sort of, the main socialising is the bar rather than ...
>
> (Gary, GM3)

Yet these public spaces, gay bars and clubs, were also, at times, felt by most of the gay men to be restrictive and encouraging of the same social practices as the strongly 'macho' environment described above:

> I think gay men are generally out and about more than straights [...] I suppose it's healthy that you go out and not stay in on your own and wallow in your own problems. It's healthy that you go out and be with your friends, but it's not too healthy in the other way because you're having alcohol, cigarettes, drugs, you know and maybe getting in a drunken state that you don't know what you're doing when you go home with someone.
>
> (David, GM1)

These alternative, safe spaces were also not clearly bounded and this created tensions. This had implications for social practices that may affect health and well-being:

> What really pisses us off is that if you are in a gay venue and there is a straight couple opposite you with their tongues down each other's throat. If we went into Yates's Wine Lodge and done that we'd either get beat up or chucked out. If you're in a gay venue you should respect it, the same as we respect it if we're in a straight venue. And that really does piss me off. The times I've nearly got in a fight through that, you know, the times I've been pulled away.
>
> (Edward, GM2)

This viewing of space as 'territory' could be seen to support previous work by Castells (1983) who suggests that 'gay ghettos' (in San Francisco) were not so much about making gay identity coherent and visible but were an extension of masculine domination through a desire to master space. These are not necessarily mutually exclusive, and from the descriptions here it seems that the creation of such spaces, and the disputes over them, are also clearly linked to the need to claim a distinct identity *and* resist the incursion of a heterosexual hegemony. As Connell (1992) has noted, to claim homosexual identity does not necessitate losing all masculine identity and the privileges that this entails.

Marginalization of non-normative bodies is not merely representational; it becomes literally built into structures and systems and has direct material consequences. All the disabled men interviewed had encountered numerous problems with physical access to buildings, even those specifically for use by people with impairments, with negative psycho-emotional consequences being implicit and sometimes explicit in such narratives:

> We actually went up to the job centre, well we couldn't actually get into the job centre cause the Disability Officer was upstairs! [...] They actually came down and discussed my case in front of everyone, I couldn't believe it, couldn't believe it.
>
> (Ron, DM3)

The message given to the disabled men was that they did not constitute the 'norm' and examples were given of how this restricted access to leisure, education and work opportunities. As well as having to deal with the psycho-emotional consequences of this, the marginalization of non-normative, impaired bodies, even by health services designed to meet these needs, could also lead to further physiological bodily breakdown:

> It's awful, for four years I've been trying to get sat straight in a wheelchair. I said to the system, to the physios, to the OTs, to the people who make the cushions, I need a cushion what's gonna level me off. 'Well you need to get your chair first Vernon, when you get

your chair we can sort the cushion out.' So I said 'No, you sort the cushion out first, I can get a wheelchair made that will take whatever sized cushion you're gonna give me.' So for coming on nearly four years I've never sat level, so it's knackered me back even worse. Because I'm always sat with a twist so me back's got an S in it now, me spine's got an S in it, according to the specialist [. . .] *We've moved a long way, but if you're not what you would call one of the norm, don't fit into that 80 per cent, you are still living in the dark ages.*

(Vernon, DM4, emphasis added)

Normative bodily representations act, then, to impact on the movement of bodies in place and space and this in turn can affect experiential and physiological embodiment. In order to explicate further the relationship between material and representational aspects of embodiment and their relationship to gender and health this section will finish by considering these issues in the context of work, paid employment.

Working bodies

Many writers continue to point out that, in contemporary Western society, men are defined by what they do, and that this is specifically conflated with what paid employment in the public sphere they undertake (for example, Petersen 1998: 49; Lee and Owens 2002: 70). This, of course, links to representations of men's bodies, discussed earlier, as objectified instruments used to fulfil these roles. Yet for the men interviewed their relationship with work was often not represented in these terms; rather, it was an experientially embodied relationship:

I come home from work and have at least two pints a night when I finish work to calm down you know. I used to work at the casino as well, used to finish there about 2 o' clock in the morning, I'd come home and it was like 4 or 5 o'clock before I could go to bed because you're buzzing, on that much of an high, you know your adrenaline, you need to come home and just calm down. If I went straight to bed I wouldn't be able to get to sleep.

(Hugh, CABS2)

In this sense, men's engagement with the everyday world of work, a definitive part of pragmatic embodiment, was also fully part of experiential embodiment ('buzzing' and 'high') and was *felt* as having some effect on underlying physiological processes (adrenaline). Whilst the importance of work as a contributor to self-esteem and therefore health remained, and was particularly strong for some men, changing employment patterns certainly raised questions for the men about the representation of 'man-as-provider' and this was seen as becoming less central to identity for most of the men.

> SR: Do you think being out of work would [adversely affect your health]?
>
> Martin: Oh God yeah. I wouldn't be out of work to be honest, I would find a job be it, just working in a local kitchen, just to keep me amused, keep occupied. I couldn't not be in work. [. . .] I think you just get low self-esteem to be honest, you'd just become depressed, really down, I think to be employed is, it gives you a certain confidence in life doesn't it, it makes you feel wanted.
>
> [. . .]
>
> SR: But for men of the older generation, what you were saying before about being out of work would that have held true for them?
>
> Martin: More in that generation than now I would have thought. Cause the men were the providers, weren't they? Whereas it's not, I suppose it is still seen as the man does the most providing for the family, but certainly the balance has levelled a little bit, hasn't it really? Women are expected to go out and work. They have to, to get the large mortgages that everyone has got nowadays, so you have to do it.
>
> (Martin, CABS3)

In this way the requirement for less physical labour and more flexible working patterns in late modernity is possibly reducing the importance of work in the construction of hegemonic *male* identity, although not its importance in overall identity construction, as identity becomes constructed as much through consumption as through production. Employment becomes 'healthy' (and conversely unemployment 'unhealthy') because self-esteem is gained as much through an actively consuming body as it is through a productive, working body:

> Some people care about themselves and their health, some don't. I think the people who don't care about their health is probably the people who are not with anyone or have no money, no job, things like that, so circumstances as well. If you've got no money, you can't buy the stuff and look after yourself, and if you're not working you've got no money.
>
> (David, GM1)

For some of the gay men in particular, paid work was only significant to the extent that it provided the finances necessary to enjoy leisure time; that is, to consume a 'gay lifestyle':

I think seriously that a lot of gay men, and women, their lives are so geared up for socializing that a lot of them go out to work just to be able to socialize more. [town] is a prime example. You'll see people from November till Easter out and about all the time, then suddenly they'll vanish off the scene, you might just see them occasionally because they're working like 24–7, to save up money through the season.

(Wayne, GM6)

This is not of course to suggest that there is only one gay lifestyle, but rather, as Forrest (1994) points out, it highlights how gay identities have become centred to some extent around the commercial scene in late modernity and the 'pink pound' has become a significant part of consumer culture.

Yet these wider changes to working patterns, a shift away from defining manhood through work, were also identified among the non-gay men interviewed. Commitment to working remained strong, but the majority of men felt that these changes acted to provide greater flexibility and freedom to change work and see it as a means to an end rather than an end in itself. Thus, when experiential embodiment suggested that physiological processes were being too adversely affected by work environments, then men frequently took responsibility for changing this situation, usually by changing job or place of work within a company:

Francis: Yeah, I left there in December, it just wasn't working out and I was going home and getting headaches and I got back to the [different work] section and was fine again, getting back to doing what I like doing.
SR: So that was a definite decision that you made to change back?
Francis: Oh yeah, yeah. Really cause I was coming home and I was like . . . just wasn't good at all. I was just always tired and got headaches and all that sort of stuff, you know.

(Francis, CABS1)

Five of the CABS and four of the gay men changed work for similar reasons during the period of the fieldwork and Bob highlights these changing attitudes well when describing what happened after a new manager arrived at his place of work:

She was very aggressive, a loud mouth, for the type of job she was doing and you don't need to be, you need to be calm and steady. I mean she was very aggressive towards me all the time. And I just said to her, 'Perhaps you're not explaining yourself properly to me, what you want me to do and things like that.' In the end we parted on bad terms [laugh] but I just thought, well at the moment with all what's going on and what's happening with me, I don't need this. So I just, I found another job, left on the Monday I think, and started the new job on the Tuesday. Cause it was pathetic, it was getting a bit silly.

(Bob, CABS6)

Yet the employment patterns found amongst the men were also affected by combinations of normative and physiological embodiment. As the men's vignettes show, three out of the six disabled men and two out of the four men with chronic illnesses were not in paid employment and the three disabled men in paid employment all worked within some aspect of the 'disability industry'. This suggests, as others have highlighted (Sapey 2000; Roulstone 2002), that despite technological changes there remains an absence of 'enabling employment' for those with impairments. Reintegrating into the work environment for the two disabled men with acute acquired impairments was often problematic but central to regaining a positive self-identity:

The respect I've got now, is much more addictive to the respect I had then [through associating with drug dealers]. Because I've earned the respect with the work that I've done, and I've got recognition throughout the County, throughout the City Council, not just working in [place] but also now as a training co-ordinator. And everybody knows me now, and are asking for me. And so I've got that respect.

(Peter, DM1)

Yet work was also felt to have an ambivalent effect on health and was certainly a less central priority in these men's lives:

You work all those hours and hours and hours. My friends are all workaholics. And I'm saying at the end of the day it don't mean squat I says 'because if you drop down dead they'll only go and get somebody else' you know and that's the truth. [...] I mean, you know to work 80/90 hours like I used to it's ridiculous.

(Ron, DM3)

It is clear that the movement of bodies through place and space both affects and is affected by aspects of (male) identities. Such movements and their fusion with identities have both positive and negative implications for health and well-being. Yet such movement is rarely a matter of free choice and structural constraints to movement often occur indirectly through hegemonic normative bodily representations being built into environments and systems. I tentatively suggest here that changing patterns of employment (production) have reduced the importance of man-as-provider representations in male identity construction and that this has generally had a positive impact for the men in terms of increasing lifestyle choices. However, this needs to be considered alongside the effects of increased consumerism on health and well-being and the fact that increasingly compressed employment opportunities and drives towards efficiency in the workplace may benefit some groups at the expense of others (Roulstone 2002).

Summary

Male embodiment should then be seen as both material and representational and while these two aspects were separated in the first two sections, this was a heuristic device employed to aid clarity rather than to suggest that they constitute separate spheres. Watson's (2000: 117) 'male body schema' provides a useful framework for exploring how these spheres may interrelate, although his overemphasis on pragmatic embodiment means that he fails to explore fully the relationships between the four elements (normative, pragmatic, experiential and visceral embodiment), and the impact of these on health and well-being for men, in his own work.

What emerges here when these relationships are more fully explicated is empirical support for recent theoretical calls to bring the biological back in to an embodied sociology of health and illness without reducing the body to the anatomical and/or physiological alone (Williams 2002; Williams 2003; Williams et al. 2003). In line with thinking on the importance of critical realist insights into health and the body (Williams 2003), the approach taken here moves beyond most previous work that considers men's bodies *either* as distinct physical entities *or* as discursive constructions. The men interviewed were both implicitly and explicitly aware of the 'real', 'fleshy' nature of (their) bodies and of physiological processes that maintained them (or not) in 'working order'. They further recognized that such physiological processes were often taken-for-granted, hidden from view. Yet, the men were also implicitly and explicitly concerned with the way (their) bodies were (re)presented and the implications of this for health practices and outcomes. These two elements, physicality and representation, were often linked or made visible through experiential embodiment, through how the men felt and experienced various aspects of their daily life. Experiential embodiment thus becomes a critical site for recognizing and understanding the emergent properties of physiological processes and also the health effects and impacts of bodily representations: that is, men's embodied experiences can provide insight into the particular conditions and contexts that create or sustain particular health practices and outcomes.

More will be said in Chapter 5 about health screening and the male body, and the particular implications of this for engagement with health services and health promotion practices generally. In the next chapter I shall begin to explore the nature of the men's relationships and the impact of these on aspects of health and well-being.

Key points

- Biological and individual behavioural explanations regarding men and health, proffered by health professionals, often fail to recognize the significance of pragmatic embodiment to men.
- Men can and do listen and learn from their own and others' bodily experiences and often adjust daily routines/practices (pragmatic embodiment) accordingly.
- Men feel a tension, linked to male identity, between a desire to have a 'good' body (tall, lean, muscular) and not wanting to be seen to be paying attention to appearance.
- Representation of male identity based on active, strong bodies becomes problematic if changes such as impairment or chronic illness make this difficult to sustain.
- Male body image was often associated with being 'macho' or 'laddish', which in turn was integrally tied to particular, potentially detrimental, health practices.
- Healthy (male) bodies are as much the product of healthy public places and policies as they are of individual behaviour(s).
- Groups of men, including gay and disabled men, can become marginalized from particular public places marked out as gendered spaces and this has material impact on health and well-being.

Key points for practice

- Those interested in improving the health of men should focus more on the lived body in everyday life rather than just on the physiological body and physiological health and well-being.
- Men have more than just a mechanistic view of their bodies. Health professionals should encourage and explore men's experiences of how they learn from and listen to their own body. This will provide good opportunities for facilitating change and positively impact on men's health and daily lives.
- Understanding how men keep healthy means recognizing how particular places and spaces become 'gendered'. Health professionals

need to understand better how 'healthy practices' are facilitated or inhibited in specific places and spaces in order to influence more positively men's health.

4 Men, relationships, emotions and health

Introduction

The issues of embodiment discussed in the previous chapter are made particularly apparent in the relationships that men have – in the way that they interact with others in everyday life. The philosophical separation of the mind from the body (Cartesian dualism), discussed at the outset of the previous chapter, is also said to have significant impact on men's emotional lives, on the way they do or do not relate to and communicate with those around them. Such dichotomous thinking has been responsible for associating men with the mind (and therefore reason) and women with the body (and therefore emotionality). This historical legacy, it is argued, leaves men either unwilling or, even if willing, struggling to experience or give expression to their emotions. As Seidler (1994: 19) states:

> As men we learn to live a lie. We learn to live *as if* we are 'rational agents' in the sense that we live beyond nature. We learn to live as if our emotional lives do not exist, at least as far as the 'public world' is concerned [...] We learn to live in our minds as the source of our identities. If we had our way as men it would be that our emotional lives did not exist at all.
>
> (emphasis in original)

Due to this historical legacy, it is argued, men's lived experience currently revolves around what has been termed 'instrumental reason' (that is, thinking and doing) at the expense of emotional expression (that is, feeling) (Seidler 1994; Bennett 1995). Likewise, work on men, social capital and health has highlighted how men's relationships are often predicated on such instrumentality to the detriment of emotional needs (Sixsmith and Boneham 2001). Yet, Cartesian dualism served not only to separate the mind and body in Western thought but also encouraged the individualization of these aspects of life; the body and the mind belonged to, or became situated within, the individual. In this way, it is understandable that 'emotions', through the nineteenth and twentieth centuries, increasingly became the province of the psy-scientists (psychologists, psychoanalysts, psychiatrists) whose focus was on the individual context of emotion development and expression (Parker et al. 1995: 12*ff*). Yet, as Williams (2001: 132) outlines, emotions are necessarily complex, multidimensional and multifaceted combining biological and cultural components and arising or emerging *within socio-relational contexts*. Feminist and postmodernist perspectives have also recently been key in questioning such apparent distinctions between mind and body. This has opened up debates on the relationship between desire and reason, corporeal intimacies and the role of 'lived experience', subjectivity, in epistemology (Williams and Bendelow 1998b: xvi).

This chapter explores the context of men's relationships, and through this the role of emotions in identity construction and management, and the impact of these on health practices. The first section looks at men's intimate,[1] long-term, sexual partnerships and begins the argument that it is antithetical to separate the instrumental from the emotional if we are to understand how men's relationships impact on health practices. The second section considers men's non-intimate relationships (those with parents, siblings, friends) and furthers the argument that emotion needs to be understood as action/active and, in this way, embodied. The third brief section considers the impact of this argument for 'action orientated emotionality' on the relationship to mental health concerns and service access for men.

Men, intimacy and health

The correlation of intimate heterosexual relationships (often operationalized as marriage) to both the self-reporting of 'good health' (Arber and Cooper 2000) and lower mortality rates in men (Gardner and Oswald 2002) in the UK is well established, as is the significance of relationship breakdown in suicide for men (Cantor and Slater 1995; Kposowa 2000). This section considers the emotional and instrumental aspects of intimate relationships and in doing so demonstrates how these are related, through aspects of gendered identity, to specific health practices and concludes by suggesting that an emotional/ instrumental dichotomy may not be sustainable.

Understanding the 'quiet man'

Intimate relationships are often towards the top of the list when men are asked what contributes (both positively and negatively) to their health and well-being and emotions represent one medium through which intimate relationship experiences are transformed into health outcomes:

> *SR:*   One of the things I'm keen to look at is whether you feel relationships have a positive or negative effect on your health or can they have either?

Martin: I think all relationships are really positive. Yeah, I'd say all relationships are positive, they give you a buzz don't they? I think that induces good health almost, it's like the sun they say that makes you feel that, it's that kind of spring feeling.

(Martin, CABS3)

And conversely for Dan who had in the last year experienced the break up of a six year long relationship:

Dan: The person who suffers is the person who doesn't expect it. So I'm the person who didn't expect it this time [...] That does affect your health, absolutely it affects your health, mentally immediately and then physically over time, because your life has to change and it first shocks your mind and then it shocks your body, that's how I see it.

SR: And do you think those two are very much inter-related?

Dan: Yeah, healthy mind, healthy body, that kind of attitude yeah, that's how I see it. Cause immediately when you lose something, or someone, it affects you physically because you lose weight or ... I don't know, some people go grey, some people lose their hair, some people whatever, you know its shock.

(Dan, CABS7)

Emotions can be seen here to consist of both experiential and physiological components that are irreducible one to the other yet intimately entwined (Williams 2001: 132). In addition, both the experience of the emotion (Martin's 'Spring feeling') and its physiological components (Dan's weight loss) can be classed as, or seen as generative of, health outcomes. What is also apparent from both these quotes is that emotions are at once embodied and formed and reformed within intersubjective encounters (Crossley 1998). Following on from the last chapter, encounters in the social world are experienced in and through the body and recognized as having physiological effects, and emotions are an integral part of this transformative process.

Despite recognizing the key role of intimate relationships in contributing to health outcomes, there were only four examples in the data of emotional confiding in such partnerships. For the one disabled man and one CABS who commented, there seemed to be a focus on what they received (emotionally) from these exchanges rather than what they gave: 'Personally I would talk about anything with my partner, I wouldn't, there's nothing that she'd ever want me to keep quiet, keep to myself, and I would always talk about it' (Owen, CABS5).

Work by Seidler (1994) and Morgan (1992), amongst others, suggests that men are action rather than communication orientated. Intimacy therefore is something demonstrated, for example through 'working for the family', rather than something spoken about. Hearn (1993) has taken this further to suggest that men are emotional but they direct their emotions into work and the wider public sphere. In this way, household emotional labour, like domestic labour, may become seen as something that men should benefit from rather than contribute to (Lupton 1998: 128). Such asymmetry regarding emotional giving in intimate heterosexual relationships has previously been noted in research by Duncombe and Marsden (1993, 1998). They suggest this could, in part, be due to a failure to recognize the different ways that men and women perform emotion work. They further suggest that men's emotional labour is often directed towards resisting emotional expression and suppressing worries and anxieties within intimate relationships, although, as Owen's quote above makes clear, the latter is not the case for all men. It seems, then, that although there is a welcome (at least rhetorically) recognition amongst the men of the move to democratize domestic and paid work within intimate relationships (see Chapter 3), the same process of democratizing emotional labour was not (even rhetorically) evidenced from the men's accounts.

This asymmetry was not the case for a gay couple interviewed, who presented a more egalitarian view of emotional exchange:

SR: What you were saying about talking, I mean there's a lot of talk about men not being able to talk.

Wayne: Yeah, I mean a lot of men it's, call it a feminine side or whatever they wanna call it, but if I have a problem or something's wrong, I speak to Andrew. I tell him something's wrong or not right, and equally he does with me. You need to have that two-way understanding. I know he's bottled things up before and I've bottled things up before. But sooner or later he'll know something's wrong and I know something's wrong with him and we talk about it and its nothing at the end of the day you know.

(Wayne, GM6)

There are a few possible explanations for this lack of data regarding emotional confiding in intimate relationships. First, it could be that the nature of this project's focus, and the interview process itself, failed to provide sufficient space for the men to present such examples of emotional exchange facilitating more 'public' than 'private' accounts (Cornwell 1984). Second, it could be that the men did not want to make public such intimate confiding, providing an example of the resisting- and suppressing-type male emotional work highlighted by Duncombe and Marsden (1998) and one man's response to a conversation about sharing personal experiences suggested as much:

> I would never tell anybody out of the family something about my family, never. I'd never do it. Some men would, and some men have to me, they've told me things about their family, but I never would. Your family is your family and that's it, nobody comes within.
>
> (Frank, DM6)

Third, whilst relationships were clearly seen as highly significant in terms of health and well-being, it could be that emotional confiding was not the element of relationships that made them significant. Research by Walker and Kushner (1999: 53) shows that boys look to female friends from an early age as a way to 'escape the ritualised banter of his mates and indulge in prolonged conversation'. In this sense, it seems likely that emotional confiding certainly plays a role in intimate relationships for men though this may not be acknowledged, or consciously recognized, as the element of the relationship that leads to positive health and well-being, with the men preferring to highlight instrumental, action-based, reasons discussed later in this section.

Intimacy, breakdown and identity

The interviews with men who had separated or divorced does suggest that loss of such intimacy can (re)create a sense of loneliness and (emotional) isolation that recent research (Frosh et al. 2002: 58) indicates is commonly present among boys. As Dan explains:

> Living on your own as well, that does make a huge difference [to health]. I mean the fact that you've got no-one to pat you on the back, no-one to pep you up, no-one to motivate you, you are completely, just you, that's it. You've got nothing. I mean you've got friends outside, and family, but you're generally on your own, living on your own. I think it's a big thing for a lot of people.
>
> (Dan, CABS7)

In this way, men perhaps often rely on female partners to provide ontological security, their sense of self, in a way that cannot be provided, or not in the same way, by other family members and friends. Whilst men may find identity through group friendships prior to long-term relationships (this is discussed more in the following section), relationship breakdown seems to create a sense of *existential angst* requiring a (re)consideration of identity. This same state is also recognized by health professionals and can even represent a form of 'medical emergency' situation:

> I had a newly registered man who turned up for his medical and was in an anxiety state. It was a medical emergency really because he

certainly was a potential risk to himself cause he was clearly distressed, very anxious. I think he'd just had a marital breakdown just the day before and needed quite a lot of input. He needed to see a doctor. We sort of counselled him there and then. The doctor obviously gave him something to try and reduce his anxiety state as an emergency situation and then we got other appropriate agencies involved. He was just obviously in an acute crisis and we managed to help him get over that crisis.

(Dawn, HP5)

Work by Lynch (1977, 1985) on the 'broken heart' has shown significant increases in mortality from heart disease, and other diseases, following separation and divorce independent of numerous other commonly associated variables (such as diet, smoking, exercise, ethnicity, family history) and that this is more significant for men than women. Given that relationship breakdown is also frequently a precursor of suicide in men, it would seem that understanding the complex links between ontological insecurity and male identity following relationship breakdown is an area that would greatly benefit from further research.

Whilst relationship breakdown was certainly a time of emotional turmoil for the gay men, this did not seem to cause the same identity disruption. This is possibly because there was a perception, even expectation, amongst the gay men that intimate relationships were frequently transient and, because of this, it was seen as important to maintain friendship networks even when in long-term partnerships:

I'm happy for anybody that is in a relationship and I hope it works. But if they sort of then forget their friends you know, I think that's a bit sad because you never know when you're gonna need them. And especially in a gay relationship it might seem all right for the first two weeks and then it will probably all go pear-shaped, you know.

(Edward, GM2)

This being the case, a sense of 'belonging' or 'identifying' as a gay man seemed to continue whether in or out of a long-term intimate partnership.

For the two disabled men who had acquired impairments during long-term relationships, the challenge to (masculine) identity seemed to lead to a greater emotional depth in their relationship. As Vernon explains:

I mean since [a leg amputation from cancer], life has changed and life means probably different to what it did then. Then it just meant, more often than not it's work, going to the pub and back to work. Like most young couples will probably see a band that weekend or

> whatever the interest is. But since this has happened it sort of ... it
> makes you take a look at life and think what you're gonna get out of
> it and what you want out of it [...] I mean it's brought us closer
> together, a lot closer.
>
> (Vernon, DM4)

As noted in other research on chronic illness (Charmaz 1995), prostate
disease (Cameron and Bernardes 1998), and disability (Gerschick and Miller
1995), emotional responses at such times often raise questions for men about
gendered identity, including previous patterns of behaviour, leading to a
higher prioritizing of family ties and emotional expressiveness. This in turn
may create increased intimacy and therefore greater contentment for both
partners (see also Lorber and Moore 2002: 58, 62). However, such increased
intimacy is by no means inevitable and, as Charmaz's (1995: 282) research
also highlights, if a new valued identity cannot be achieved by men following
the onset of chronic illness or physical impairment, then intimate relationships can become strained and eventually breakdown. This situation may also
be different for gay, disabled men where the rise of 'body fetishism', a hyper-
importance attached to appearance in gay culture, creates additional difficulties for those with visible physical impairment in finding or sustaining
intimate relationships (Butler 2001; O'Neill and Hird 2001).

Intimacy and 'lifestyle'

It seems likely, then, that although emotional confiding is rarely mentioned
by men, it has a role to play in positive health outcomes that is only fully
recognized once that intimacy is no longer present; that is, after a relationship has broken down. What are highlighted by men as being beneficial to
health and well-being are 'lifestyle' changes made after entering into an
intimate relationship; what could be termed instrumental factors as they are
action rather than communication orientated. The health professionals also
give precedence to 'lifestyle' changes as the significant factor in producing
positive health outcomes for men in intimate relationships. As Collette
suggests:

> You know, you can drink, you can eat, you can smoke and do all
> these things. It's all an adolescent sort of attitude really, a cavalier
> attitude to their health really [...] I think a lot of single men take that
> cavalier attitude towards health perhaps longer than married men.
>
> (Collette, CP2)

Looking at some of these lifestyle factors specifically, just over half of the
men currently in heterosexual, long-term relationships mentioned that their

diets improved on entering the relationship. This concurs with other research that shows married men's diets are more in line with recommended dietary guidelines than those of single men (Roos et al. 1998). This process is graphically illustrated by Quinn:

> *Quinn:* Lucy is very healthy, she eats all the right things, she drinks prune juice (laugh). She is really health conscious and she makes sure that I eat the right things. She's a vegetarian so I hardly ever get meat. Basically she eats quorn right, so I eat quorn cause I can't see the point of buying one thing for one and one for the other.
>
> *SR:* Yeah, so you eat healthily but that's because Lucy does most of the preparation?
>
> *Quinn:* Yeah. I'll tell you a funny story. When she first moved in here me and my brother lived here. And we used to eat one loaf of bread *each* with our tea. And we had chips every night, proper chips, every night. So we'd have chips and egg, or chips and beans or . . . and one loaf of bread every meal we used to eat. We had our breakfast in the morning then we didn't have any dinner and we'd have tea and it would be chips and summit and a loaf of bread each. We just used to eat it and never think about it, just get it down our neck like.
>
> [Quinn, DM2]

Yet it was not *only* being in a long-term, heterosexual relationship that was a significant factor in pursuing a 'healthy' diet. As highlighted in the previous chapter, for those men concerned with idealized male body image, dietary care is an integral part of the process of achieving this. Also chronic illness and physical impairment play a part in motivating men to consider their diet, as the following quotations indicate:

> I'm pleased to say I haven't really suffered from the diabetes for a good while. You know even though she's [wife] gone, I've got myself a great cleaner who cooks me a meal and brings it with her, a proper meal. Because she does this, because she cooks me good meals, I don't get ill with my diabetes which is really, really important. Cause it's the last thing I need to do at this moment in time when I've got to look after everything.
>
> (Larry, CABS4)

> I know what to eat and what not to eat, I'd read the back of the packet, tells you how much fat's in it and I try and keep my fat right down. Saturated fat particularly because of the MS [Multiple Sclerosis], I always look at the saturated fat content of anything.
>
> (Bob, CABS6)

> I'm a bit overweight, but it's hard when you're in a chair to try and keep your weight down no matter what exercises you do. And it's not a matter of just trying to eat the right food, you do try and eat the right food 'cause you play sport, you've got to eat the right food. You can't just go and fill yourself full of pie and chips everyday. Though you love em.
>
> (Vernon, DM4)

Although these men are obviously aware of their need for specific dietary regimens, as Larry's quotation illustrates, gendered expectations still mean that men often, though not always, appropriate women to ensure these 'domestic' dietary needs are met.

There was a lack of comment regarding diet in all but one of the gay men's interviews. Whilst there is now a great deal written about the 'politics of food' within family units (for example, Charles and Kerr 1988; Travers 1996), such work seems lacking within non-nuclear couples and/or units. This is clearly an area that would benefit from further research to ascertain if long-term gay relationships bring similar dietary changes to heterosexual relationships.

Changes in alcohol consumption were also a significant factor in long-term relationships. Unlike dietary changes, the men often linked these narratives to fatherhood as much as to relationships *per se*:

> I was one of the beer-swilling types not that long ago. But now things change and we [as a couple] enjoy ourselves still, but we enjoy ourselves wanting to know that we are able to put up with any emergency that may occur. We take it easy until she's [the baby] of an age where she can look after herself.
>
> (Owen, CABS6)

This seems to be representative of a more general 'settling down' and 'responsibility' narrative (see also Chapter 2) following becoming a father that primarily relates to a reduction in going out to bars, pubs, particularly with 'mates', and therefore a reduction in drinking to excess (see also Lewis 1986). This reduction in high levels of alcohol consumption following settling into a long-term relationship is supported by evidence from the General Household Survey (GHS)(Office of National Statistics 2000) with married men being far less likely to consume above recommended daily limits (36 per cent) than single (never married) men (47 per cent). Evidence for the positive effects of fathering on alcohol consumption is lacking, with married fathers being marginally more likely (38 per cent) to consume above recommended amounts than married men without children (34 per cent).

For the gay men in long-term partnerships, similar narratives of 'settling down' were also present, again relating as much to reducing going out as to reducing drinking:

> I certainly don't go out drinking, partly because I don't enjoy drinking anyway as much because I'm getting older [laugh], but I just don't go out drinking as much as I used to. I mean I used to go out at least three or four times a week before I met [name], now we're lucky if we go out once a week.
>
> (Gary, GM3)

Whilst the men's accounts relating to physical activity, exercise and sport are covered in detail elsewhere (Robertson 2003), it is worth noting here that the association of these as health practices to men's relationships was contradictory. There was some feeling that settling into marriage and/or fathering reduced opportunities for what some health professionals see as one of the few 'healthy behaviours' that men engage in:

> It [marriage] often does mean that with other commitments they might cut down on what I'd perceive to be their only area of health promotion, which is the exercise. It often means you don't have time for going out and doing it.
>
> (John, HP3)

> It's just finding time, family life's obviously a priority. I've got other things to deal with. The sport, other than playing a game of golf this last month, I've not played ... I used to play squash and I used to play football, but it's just time really. It must be two or three years now since I've had a game of football but it's only a year since I had a game of squash. I used to play every week. It's a good workout and I will start that again one day it's just finding time to fit it all in.
>
> (Owen, CABS5)

There was also a strong relationship made between 'sporting friendships', 'macho' characteristics and associated negative health practices:

> I think the culture is still for a lot of exercise is done as a group activity with your friends and then its followed on maybe by heavy drinking session or it might be associated with going out and then people are smoking.
>
> (John, HP3)

SR: So traditional masculinity is?

Neil: Is going to the pub, drinking 20 pints of larger with your mates after a game of football, and going for a curry, basically . . .

(Neil, GM5)

Yet, for other men, the process of becoming a father was recognized as something that kept them mentally and physically alert and active:

Frank: I think the kids have a relationship with everything I do because my whole life's geared round them. They certainly have an effect on me health. I mean if I just sat here everyday, not playing with the kids, or taking them out, I'd be a lot worse. Because I think if you sat there all the time just gawping at the telly, you're gonna stiffen up anyway, even the average person will stiffen up.

SR: So the kids make sure that you get out?

Frank: Yeah definitely. The kids just wouldn't let you stay in every single day with them and sit there; they'd be pulling your hair out and everything [laugh].

(Frank, DM6)

Once again, we see here that the love and care (emotions) Frank obviously has for his children is seen, demonstrated, or made apparent through physical action.

The men's accounts show no clear evidence regarding relationships and smoking, with the only references to having stopped being related to managing chronic illness, although Larry also links stopping smoking directly to fatherhood and potentially detrimental health outcomes:

So, yeah, my little boy obviously made a world of difference to me and to the way I act. Like I say, the stopping smoking, that is a big part of the health plan. Wasn't for money, wasn't for anything else, basically it's so I wouldn't be sat wheezing on the park bench while my little boy was playing football. Might not play football with him, but I can . . . Cause I mean most diabetics I know who smoked at the rate I did were losing limbs and things already.

(Larry, CABS4)

For the gay men an additional 'lifestyle' factor given great importance when thinking about intimate relationships and health was 'safe(r) sex' through monogamy. Issues of trust and honesty were of key importance here as anal-genital sex without a condom often becomes symbolic of the love and intimacy expected of a long-term partner as the following conversation suggests (see also Bloor 1995):

SR: What things would you say have the most positive benefit for yourselves in terms of staying well?

Andrew: Monogamy, yeah. We said from day one, before we got together, if there was ever a point in the relationship where either of us felt the need to go off with somebody else we'd talk about it first and then come to a decision of what was happening. Not do it and then come back and say, 'I've got something to tell you' because it's too late then anyway.

Wayne: But then from people we know and what we see, the gay scene is very sort of scatty. One minute somebody meets somebody and within five minutes they are so in love with that person, they've met the 'right' person. The following day they're in tears. The following night, 'Oh I've met somebody.' And you're like but ... I mean fortunately me and Andrew don't have that type of relationship. He knows all my past relationships, I know all his, and nobody can jump out of the woodwork and put a spanner in that and so we trust each other.

(Andrew and Wayne, GM6&7)

The difficulty of this is that there can be complacency where gay men believe they are safe *because of* the intimate relationship and a possible overestimating of a partner's fidelity (Connell et al. 1993: 123).[2] Love, sexual activity and risk need to be negotiated within intimate gay partnerships and this is an ongoing and complex task (Rhodes and Cusick 2000).

It seems apparent that, although the emotional and instrumental aspects of intimate relationships have been presented separately, they are clearly integrated. The notions of trust, responsibility and care highlighted, and how these relate to issues of identity, suggest that health practices ('lifestyle' factors) are not independent of social contexts that are emotionally experienced. Rather, the emotions invested and experienced in such relationships are made apparent instrumentally, through actions, and this process currently remains gendered. For example, the changes in married men's diets can be interpreted as the action product of feminized 'care'; the reduction in going out and alcohol consumption can be understood as the practical expression of a masculine idea(l) of 'responsibility' or 'commitment' within intimate relationships; penetrative sex may be the embodied representation of both love and trust given the potential risks involved, particularly for gay men (and women). In this sense, emotions are purposive (Crossley 1998), being represented both as and in actions, including those that become (re)classified as health practices.

Wider relationships, men and health

It is relatively commonplace to highlight the (emotionally) poor nature of men's relationships, particularly those with other men (Miller 1992; Seidler 1992), to the point where this has (almost) become an accepted wisdom. This section examines men's non-intimate relationships (those with parents, siblings and friends) continuing the work begun in the previous section in highlighting the interplay between emotions and gendered identity and how this impacts on health and well-being. In doing so, I further the following arguments: firstly, that emotional investment in men's relationships is often, though not exclusively, recognized instrumentally, as activity/activities, rather than as communicative expressions of feeling; and, secondly, that because of this, emotions cannot be understood as detached from the gendered, socio-relational contexts in which they occur.

Supporting families?

One of the first things that stands out when considering the men's narratives about relationships is the importance that continues to be attached to parents, particularly mothers, by the men. Given the age range of the men (27–43 years) it is clearly significant that 12 of the men provided unsolicited accounts of support being provided in times of need by parents (five other men had mothers who had passed away or were currently unwell). This support was both emotional and practical (instrumental) as the following quotations highlight:

> I've lost friends and everything you know over in Ireland [when in the Army]. That really ... the first time I went to Ireland, when I come home on leave I was quiet, then I broke down. I'd seen someone ... and it really got to me like. I think I was crying for two days solid to me mum and dad and everything.
>
> (Hugh, CABS2)

> I mean when I came out [of hospital], I couldn't bath myself, do anything for myself. And we ended up ... well me father had to go up to the local hospital and they told him, my dad, just to take what he needed because there was nothing available whatsoever for me at home, there was literally nothing.
>
> (Ron, DM3)

Such narratives regarding the importance of parents and parental support for men were totally absent from the health professionals' narratives (as they often are in the wider 'men's health' literature) indicating that such input often goes unrecognized. The idea that parental caring work (predominantly carried out by mothers) goes unrecognized is far from new (see Clarke and Popay 1998) but the identification of the continuing role of parental support for men in this age group, and its contribution to health and well-being, would certainly seem a fruitful and necessary area for future research.

Mothers featured particularly significantly as emotional confidants for the gay men, identified in this way by six out of the seven, being representative of an ongoing form of support rather than just being present in crisis situations. However, there were no examples of the gay men engaging in a similar level of intimacy with their fathers and two of the gay men made it clear that their sexuality posed a specific problem for their relationships with their fathers. As David explains:

> I'm very, very close to my Mum, she's disabled and I'm very close to her, we talk two or three times a week on the phone and we're very close. If I have any problems, any secrets, or any concerns or worries I would speak to her about it. Erm, my father and I don't really get on well. That's because he doesn't like gay people, so that includes me. I keep trying to say to him that I'm not gonna change, it's the way I am, I love you as my father and I want you to love me as your son. I think, I think he does love me but he obviously shows that he doesn't like the gay bit, but that's his problem, even though it's my problem because it affects me.
>
> (David, GM1)

Clearly, the role of homophobia in the construction of (hegemonic) male identity can make it inimical even for loving fathers to get emotionally close to their gay sons (Cramer and Roach 1988) and this was identified by these gay men as having a potentially detrimental effect on well-being.

Fathers did feature as providers of support (both emotional and instrumental) in the narratives of some disabled men and CABS. Ron's narrative below highlights how the (re)negotiation of a disabled, male identity after acquiring a physical impairment is not something that happens in isolation but requires (re)negotiation of wider family relations including, significantly for him, those with his father:

> I must admit I've got a better relationship with me father since the disability because ... well he's a man's man should we say. And because he's seen me go from working quite a lot of hours and doing exactly what he did, having two children and a house, a family and a car, you know the proper so called correct thing. To suddenly being ... I couldn't feed myself, my wife changed me, she fed me, toileted

> me. *And he had to help.* And seeing his son suddenly going from one
> to this, his attitude certainly changed. And we've got more of a
> personal um, definitely a personal bonding more ... not like son and
> dad but more personal and more loving even. I mean even at my age,
> you could say a more loving relationship, more than just 'oh he's me
> dad' type of thing.
>
> (Ron, DM3, emphasis added)

As highlighted in the previous section, the negotiation of a disabled
(male) identity may result in an increased need and/or desire to communicate, challenging previous hegemonic male patterns of emotional passivity.
However, this new emotional depth or 'personal bond' that has developed
between Ron and his father has done so *through, and because of, engagement in
instrumental, practical tasks*, not independently of them. This has resonance
with the way that midwives encourage instrumental, practical interaction
between mothers (though often not fathers to the same extent) and their
newborn babies in order to achieve 'maternal bonding', the process of emotional attachment.

Such support from parents and wider family was not available to all men
and seemed particularly absent if a mother was no longer actively present
either through death or ill-health:

> The thing is, cause I'm a bloke and it's the way I've been [helpful], I
> tend to hold everyone else up. But when I need it they're not around.
> [...] it's like you give out so much to other people, and they know
> you need help, but they just don't take notice. The brother-in law
> knows I need this doing, but where is he to do it? It's all right when
> he wants me to help him but he's not fucking here to help me. I
> don't like to come out and say, 'I need this doing', I think they
> should understand the predicament me and the wife's in [...] I've got
> two sisters and a brother, be lucky if they've been here half a dozen
> times between all three of them [since the amputation]. I don't think
> they can handle it [...] All I get off me brother is, 'What the fucking
> hell are you doing in that chair? Why don't you get out and walk?
> Why can't you get this done, why can't you get that done?'
>
> (Vernon, DM4)

It seems Vernon clearly links the lack of practical support to a lack of
emotional care for his and his wife's 'predicament' by his wider family
members. Recent research on men, health and social capital has highlighted
how men's social ties are predicated on instrumentality to the neglect of
emotional needs (Sixsmith and Boneham 2001: 52). I would suggest, though,
that men consider instrumentality (action) not merely a form of emotional

expression but as constitutive of the emotion itself. The provision of practical help to Vernon and his wife *is* love and care rather than just its representation or expression. *For men, emotion is integrated into action.* Harré (1991: 142*ff*) and Merleau-Ponty (1971) take a similar view that emotions refer not to what someone is, or feels, but to what someone does: 'Anger, shame, hate and love are not psychic facts hidden at the bottom of another's consciousness: they are types of behaviour or styles of conduct which are visible from the outside' (Merleau-Ponty 1971: 52).

Yet, this is not divorced from its gendered context and it is the men (brother and brother-in-law) that Vernon sees as mainly responsible for not recognizing and certainly for not providing this practical support and thus demonstrating their lack of (emotional) care.

Healthy friendships

For many of the men, friendship was frequently equated with 'getting out', often associated with drinking in pubs, bars, clubs. 'Getting out' was not just about physical place but seemed also to be about 'escape' or 'release' from aspects of daily life (usually termed 'stress') into specifically masculine space:

Dan: The important part of men's lifestyles from what I've seen, is the need to escape reality through how they live. And that in turn is shown through, or displayed through, what they wear, what they drink, where they go, what activities they take up and their general attitude at that time.

SR: Can you give me any examples?

Dan: Well, in your 20s you have your going to the pub and getting smashed with your mates, that's escape. Then into your 30s perhaps like not just alcohol, drugs as I say, and relationships where there's not much thought about it, its just kind of like ready-made relationship at the weekend and then off you go again the weekend later. That kind of lifestyle, promiscuous really on every angle, which is going to affect you physically and mentally somewhere down the line. It's like a time bomb.

(Dan, CABS7)

Other research also seems to indicate that such use of alcohol as a means of escape is gendered and whereas women more often reported drinking to solve problems, men more frequently drank in order to gain 'hedonic benefits' (Mäkelä and Mustonen 2000). Indeed, as outlined in Chapter 2, such 'release' itself is understood by the men as being healthy, part of a balanced life. The importance of this process, drinking with friends to 'escape', should not be underestimated and was highlighted in many of the interviews as being beneficial, in terms of mental well-being, and yet potentially detrimental to physical health. Frosh et al. (2002: 60) point out that whilst young men are often said to feel a disjunction between a public, 'laddish' image and 'private self', this does not do justice to the complexity of masculine identity and 'authentic male self' is constructed in both public and private contexts. Likewise, research by Linda McDowell (2002) also indicates that masculine identities can accommodate both 'laddism' and ideal(s) of domesticity for young men.

Unquestioning acceptance into male peer friendship groups was certainly reaffirming for the men and presented as positive in terms of well-being, as Owen explains when talking about the movement between intimate relationships and friendships when he was younger:

> Yeah, it was just like getting back on board again. One of me mates went away, got married, got divorced, come back, and it's like he's never been away, never saw him for four years but when he did come back in the fold, 'All right, how you doing?' sort of thing, 'Do you want a beer?' *You don't actually support them, you do just by being a mate and involving them again.* You don't talk about it very often, it's happened and you come back and there's nothing you can do about it. It's not bad place to be, you just get over it and just get back on and everyone just has a laugh again, all single lads together.
>
> (Owen, CABS5, emphasis added)

It is important here not to overlook the fact that, whereas such peer friendship groups may be beneficial to men in terms of mental well-being, masculine identity is often (re)affirmed in such groups through misogyny, homophobia and violence that reinforces hegemonic ideals and can result in the marginalization/subordination of others – see Gough and Edwards (1998) for an example of this process in action.

The health professionals also recognized 'getting out', drinking, as an integral part of younger men's friendships as Collette highlights when describing a recent discussion with her son prior to him leaving for university:

> He said 'I couldn't go through university without a drink cause that would be stupid' you know. 'I couldn't cope with not drinking at university.' You'd have to do it. There's no way, you couldn't sort of go through university for four years and not be sort of one of the boys and get laughed at, you know.
>
> (Collette, HP2)

Such friendships were described either by the single CABS in the study or by those men in long-term relationships as something engaged in prior to entering the relationship. In this way 'going out' becomes juxtaposed to the 'settling down' narrative of intimate relationships described in the previous section. This change in the nature of men's social ties through the lifecourse – a move expressed as 'entering marriage, exiting friendships' by one researcher (Cohen 1992: 119) – has been noted in previous research on men's friendships in the US (Cohen 1992) and the UK (Sixsmith and Boneham 2001).

However, this may oversimplify the nature of men's friendships both during and beyond this transition. Friendships established through the earlier 'going out' years sometimes evolved over time, often settling into regular meetings for specific shared activities with less emphasis on hedonism:

Francis: I mean the football we've known each other since youth club, we're talking nearly 20, well the best part of 20 years now.

SR: So is there social activity linked in and around it then, you know, having a drink afterwards or . . .?

Francis: No we're all passed that a bit now I think. Some of them are a bit older than that so we can't quite do the drink afterwards anymore and besides we all drive there. A lot of them are married with kids now anyway. I mean the badminton ones, we do still see quite a lot of each other socially through people getting married and birthdays and things like that.

(Francis, CABS1)

They can also evolve through adversity, and difficult times act to provide a place for more communicative engagement although, as Dan highlights, this often runs parallel to an ongoing requirement to reaffirm (male) identity through unquestioning acceptance and hedonistic escape:

Yeah I was driven to it [socializing and drinking], more so then, to just get out and to make me forget any problems that had happened and it helps [. . .] I'm from [city] and it's difficult to get over there and just sit down and talk or go out and talk. Luckily I've got two close friends who live in this area and I became close to them when I split up with me girlfriend. They were very good and very understanding and luckily are free to go out most nights and I did a combination of the two they would counsel me and never get tired of it. And one was going through a similar thing as well so that helped enormously. So I could do the counselling and the forgetting both in one go.

(Dan, CABS7)

This evolving through adversity may not always be into deeper friendship and can sometimes lead men to move away from (hegemonic) male peer groups. For Peter, acquiring a disabled (male) identity marginalized him from previous 'laddish' friendships, leading to a (re)evaluation of what friendship is or should be:

> So I was in this [rehabilitation] home, a place where I didn't know anybody, me family and friends were back in [the town]. Me friends didn't come and see me. The friends I've got now are not the same friends that I had. Those friends in the past are all acquaintances now. I think that had an effect on me because I had nothing to get up for, nothing to look forward to [...] My worst mistake is, I thought they were still my friends, so I was going back to see them. I suppose I was still a bit naive at the time, I wasn't aware of the fact that they just basically washed their hands of me [...] And I suppose that really dawned on me, the fact that well they haven't bothered ringing, hadn't bothered coming down to see me and one thing and another.
>
> (Peter, DM1)

Again the link is between action *as* emotion. They were not 'true' friends as they made no practical effort to contact him; the lack of action *is* lack of emotional care and friendship not just its representation. A distinction between 'acquaintance' and 'true' or 'close' friendship was made by almost all the men, and the process of negotiation into a close friendship was presented by many as difficult, even risky: 'I mean men are strange beasties, they talk about, they'll just talk about general news, general items, until probably I don't know six months into it, then they might start sharing' (Bob, CABS6).

This difficulty in negotiating deeper friendships has been shown in previous theoretical and empirical work to be linked to hegemonic masculine identities based on fear of appearing vulnerable and the need to appear independent (Seidler 1992; Sixsmith and Boneham 2001). It is also undoubtedly this process that leads men to have smaller social support networks than women, having a similar number of close friendships (often, as Bob indicates above, developed over long periods) but fewer acquaintances (Wellman 1992). There was a distinct lack of emotional confiding in 'acquaintances', though not in 'true' friendships amongst the men. This differs from the confiding that women engage in with acquaintances found in other empirical work (Sixsmith et al. 2001) that will undoubtedly impact on health and well-being (Sixsmith and Boneham 2001, Sixsmith et al. 2001). As recent ESRC funded research (Arber and Davidson 2002) has shown, this desire for smaller social networks persists through the ageing process, particularly amongst divorced or never married men who have no female partner to facilitate and maintain wider social networks.

For the gay men, this process of developing closer friendships did not seem as difficult. Gay male identity, positioned in alliance with femininity and in juxtaposition to hegemonic ideas of stoicism, gave the gay men permission to be more emotionally expressive. This was seen to impact on the quality of friendships as David highlights when talking about the support he received after a relationship breakdown and contrasting this with straight men and relationship breakdown:

> Probably support would be there [for straight men] but not to the same sort of motherly degree. As gay men we are supposed to be more emotional anyway and our feelings are supposed to be stronger and things. So there probably is support there from their mates but not so cuddly, cuddly, pally, pally more ... 'Argh you'll get over it mate, there's a next shag around the corner' you know that's probably the attitude of what I know of some straight mates. That's the attitude they have.
>
> (David, GM1)

Nardi (1992: 110) suggests that friendships for gay men are often seen in a similar way to family ties in that they 'provide the role of maintaining physical and emotional well-being'. Gay men's accounts here concur with Nardi's (1992) empirical work, highlighting the importance of instrumental *and* emotional confiding in such friendships brought about through shared marginal identity and the experience of prejudice:

> I think we're closer because of the prejudice against gay people, so we've got our own little clubs. And somewhere like [town] I think there's what four, five clubs and it's only a small town so everyone knows each other [...] So I think the whole gay community sort of sticks together ... partly because of all the prejudices, but it's just something that's just happened.
>
> (Gary, GM3)

The association of gay men with femininity and thereby emotional expressiveness can give the appearance of a fixed dichotomy between emotion and instrumentality (as well as femininity/masculinity) with gay men being associated with the former and straight men with the latter. Yet, as Fee (2000) suggests, and the following narrative highlights, gay/straight relationships may blur such boundaries:

> *SR:*   Do you think straight men don't have the opportunity to talk with close friends in the same way that gay men do?
>
> *Edward:*   Probably. I mean I used to go out with a fellar that said he was straight, and his wife said 'Are you having an affair?' [laugh] If she only knew! [laugh] Yeah, but if he'd got any problems he would rather talk to me about them than he would his wife. So I don't

> know whether I feel that a gay person is more sympathetic, or easy
> to talk to, or more understanding, I don't know.
>
> (Edward, GM2)

It seems here that the emotional/instrumental polarization is hard to sustain and that the vibrant physicality of intimacy is both in sexual intercourse and confiding; that is, it provides a further example of embodied emotionality.

In concluding this section it seems overly simplistic to suggest that men's non-intimate relationships should be seen solely in instrumental, practical terms. Rather the data here suggest that the emotional/instrumental gender divide (that situates men with the latter) is not sustainable and fails to recognize the role of practical action *as actually constitutive of* emotional intimacy for men. This wrapping of relationships with issues of gendered identity has a range of implications both directly for health practices (lifestyle 'choices') and also significantly for what the men consider to be appropriate 'support' and this is considered in more detail in the following chapter.

Implications for mental health

The relationship between instrumental/(action) and communicative/(emotional) orientations have particular significance when considering issues of mental health and well-being. Issues of health service engagement are primarily dealt with in the following chapter, so it is more appropriate to consider here the lay men's narratives regarding mental health generally and access to services for mental health/well-being concerns.

In regard to distinctions between 'health' and 'illness', it was clear that there was some uncertainty amongst the men about whether issues often generically classified as 'minor mental health' (such as depression, anxiety) did actually represent an 'illness' that therefore required health professional intervention:

> There's a lot of pressure on, certainly young men 25 to 35, but why
> they don't go and see a doctor I don't know. I suppose they don't see
> it [depression] as an illness in a way. An illness is 'God me arm's sore',
> 'God I've got a sore pain in the chest'. Mental illness isn't something
> like that. I guess in a way it's almost untreatable, well it's not cause
> there's a lot of counselling. But people think or perceive that you just
> get whacked on a load of drugs and left to it. It's treating an illness
> when they don't think they are actually ill they are just a bit down at
> the moment. I don't think they perceive depression as an illness.
>
> (Martin, CABS3)

It also seemed that, unlike physical illness that represented a legitimate reason for accessing health services, to need help for what was perceived as coping with (albeit difficult) aspects of daily life still carries a stigma, and particularly so for men. As Kiaran explains when talking about stress at work:

> It's not something . . . you wouldn't go to the pub and tell your mates that you're feeling depressed. Where women would [. . .] Men are not likely to say that they're stressed at work. Perhaps it's just a man thing, that men are not supposed to suffer with stress, it's a women's thing. And even as a gay man I still think that. I mean I was off ill from work last year, I got glandular fever, and people were saying, 'Oh its stress related'. 'Its *not* bloody stress related!'
>
> (Kiaran, GM4)

Others have also noted (O'Brien et al. 2005; Emslie et al. 2006) how seeking help for depression presents men with particular challenges to masculinity. As suggested in the quotes above, there is a tendency for men especially to be unwilling to elaborate or define problems as being 'mental health' concerns and this is often related, particularly in younger men (O'Brien et al. 2005: 510), to narratives of independence, self-sufficiency, and control.

Hugh also takes up these themes in his narrative about the support available following traumatic experiences in the army:

> *Hugh:*   You had chance of going for counselling and everything, they'd give you that option.
> *SR:*   And did yourself and a lot of those blokes make use of those options?
> *Hugh:*   No. *It weren't like the manly thing to do* really. You used to talk it out between you and all help each other through it really [. . .] I know there were a lot of suicides, with a few of the guys, coming back from Ireland. They were like the loners kinds of people you know.
>
> (Hugh, CABS2, emphasis added)

Hugh also raises another significant issue here that was common to these narratives: that seeking health-service intervention for coping with traumatic aspects of life represented a safety net that should be there for those men who did not have social support available. As Dan also highlights:

> I've never thought I needed counselling for that separation with the girlfriend. I've done it really with my friends, so I never had to think about it. They put me mind to rest or led me through it, whereas, if I didn't have that, then you would need somebody. Counselling is a bit of a swear word to some people? Really it's just talking to people

> who you feel you can trust. So no I wouldn't have considered it
> unless I had nobody to talk to who I could trust.
>
> (Dan, CABS7)

In a sense, this seems to stand in contrast to the findings of O'Brien et al.
(2005) where the young men especially felt self-disclosure about emotional
issues was inappropriate for men or at least carried significant risks of ridicule.
Yet accounts here suggest that this is only part of the story. The close relationships that men can develop, outlined above and in the second section of
this chapter, do allow some scope for dealing with minor mental health
concerns through confiding but also through getting out and 'forgetting'. It
also becomes apparent that the men's constructions of such concerns as
personal, family, or social issues rather than health issues mitigate against
seeking help from health services. For many, to get professional help for such
concerns seemed to represent an impersonal approach to personal
circumstances:

> I think everybody's different, because I would never ever go to a
> counsellor, I wouldn't go and talk to a complete stranger about any
> problems I've got, no way. Cause I think it would just be a waste of
> time that's my personal opinion of it. Because as soon as you come
> out that room you're just another person, the next one goes in, and
> that's it. So if I've got a problem I'd rather go to a friend and talk it
> over with a friend.
>
> (Edward, GM2)

For other men, this construction of minor mental health problems as 'not
illness', and as being related to 'private' issues, also combined with narratives
of (hegemonic) male coping where narratives of 'getting through' or 'getting
over' such issues seemed significant in 'proving' (hegemonic) male identity:

> *SR:* If you're not feeling good, what do you do?
> *Martin:* Um, *get over it* [laugh] basically. I don't think 'right I'm feeling really
> depressed so I'm gonna raid the fridge or raid the freezer', *just get
> over it*. Go out with me mates or something or . . . yeah, I *get over it*. I
> guess just being with me mates or whatever is, take me mind off
> things and *get on with it*.
>
> (Martin, CABS3, emphasis added)

Such an approach is often presented as men ignoring or not 'dealing'
with issues, but the action orientation of this 'getting out', 'escape' and
'forgetting' seemed to provide one way out of a downward spiral into
depression with these actions themselves being presented as cathartic.

Previous theoretical work has suggested that men's 'action orientation' may explain their reluctance to engage with counselling services that are communication orientated (Bennett 1995) and 'psy' science approaches to practice based on verbal communication may fail to address the needs of men (and perhaps some women) who prefer to physically 'work through' issues or at least to use action as the starting point. With this in mind some recent projects working with men around depression have absorbed this action-orientation approach to emotional life into their work, taking men out of 'discussion' based work, at least initially, and into engagement with practical activities with some success (Melluish and Bulmer 1999; Borg 2002).

Summary

Much previous work on masculinity has highlighted the difficulties that men have in both feeling and expressing emotions, leading to 'poor' relationships at all levels, and impacting negatively on health and well-being. Such work often internalizes and individualizes 'emotion' rather than seeing it as an active force operating through and in complex sets of social relations. It also often limits what constitutes 'emotion' or 'emotional expression' to the process of 'talking through' issues, 'confiding'. In doing so this work fails to fully appreciate the role that emotions play in the construction and/or maintenance of identity and the process of transformation of embodied experience into health practices; that is, it fails to link emotion and action.

Accounts here suggest that there is a strong expectation for men's social ties to evolve (naturally) over the lifecourse, shifting from public friendships based around hedonistic pleasure (an integrally emotional state) to private coupledom based around intimacy. This process often unconsciously produces related health practices (smoking, drinking, excess through the former, and a reduction of these excesses and improved diet in the latter) and was clearly part of the men's *habitus*; their acquired set of generative dispositions (Bourdieu 1979).

Yet such (apparently natural) transitions in social ties were often disrupted by a range of forces or events. The breakdown of long-term intimate relationships destabilized male identity based on (male?) assumptions of such relations being enduring; the acquisition of physical impairment or chronic illness required (re)consideration of male identity and relationships; and identifying as 'gay' raised questions about whether transition into a 'settling-down' life phase was either achievable or even desirable. In this way, such disruptions require the (re)consideration of previous sets of generative dispositions that are integrally related to 'who we are', our ontological being. Such (re)consideration may never be fully resolved with new practical necessities and old generative dispositions struggling to be reconciled. It seems clear though that strong social ties, or ties that become developed or strengthened during such events, may help secure a valued identity and thus facilitate well-being.

For many of the men (though not to the same extent for the gay men) the development of strong social ties was integrally linked to instrumentality, practical activity. There is a propensity in the literature on men's friendships to suggest that this is a poor second to, or a polar opposite to, emotional depth and intimacy. Yet such a view suggests a failure to see emotion *as and in action* rather than separate from it. In this way, as Arber and Davidson (2002) point out: 'we tend to measure the quantity and quality of social networks with a "feminine ruler"' and different means of understanding intimacy and friendship for men need to be found. I suggest that, for men, emotional commitment is first demonstrated, shown as and in action, before it becomes safe to engage in communicative action, as Hugh highlights when describing friendships in the army:

> I mean your friends in the army are real friends. Your life depends on them, you know, and if they could do anything to help you, they would do, there's no ... It's like unconditional love really at the end of the day. You could be out on the streets and your life is in your mate's hands, you all watch each other's back. It brought you so close it was unbelievable [...] It's quite hard to explain really, you can tell these kind of guys anything and everyone would help each other and talk it over, cause they'd been through similar experiences of life.
>
> (Hugh, CABS2)

Key points

- Intimate, sexual relations are seen by men as being generative of both positive and negative health outcomes.
- These health outcomes are linked to 'feelings' but more often to changes in specific 'health practices' that occur 'naturally' on entering and exiting these relations.
- Breakdown of such relationships often creates instability and uncertainty, a sense of *existential angst*, for men which can require a (re)negotiation of their (male) identity.
- Parents, particularly mothers, continue to provide an important source of support, both practical and emotional, for men even well into their middle-age.
- It is often engagement in practical activities, tasks, either as recipient or provider, that generates deeper emotional bonds for men. Emotion is integrated into action.
- Friendships for men often change through the lifecourse, shifting

from the hedonistic 'escape' when younger to longer term relationships on 'settling down'.

- Friendships are important for men in creating the necessary conditions for confiding but also in helping with the instrumental process of 'getting out' and 'forgetting'.
- Mental health issues seemed to sit uncomfortably with the health/ill-health split that the men tried to maintain.
- The linking of action with emotion for men may mean that dealing with mental health concerns requires 'doing' rather than 'talking', at least to begin with.

Key points for practice

- Recognizing emotion *as* action is crucial in understanding how trust is developed and therefore how space for communicative action ('emotional confiding') can be created in health work with men.
- Changes in social relationships – including marriage, becoming a father, and divorce – often stimulate a renegotiation of (male) identity that provides opportunities for health-professional work with men.
- There is a need for health professionals to recognize, value and, when appropriate, use the support that men of middle age continue to receive from their parents.
- Basing therapeutic mental health work in action based rather than communication based models, at least in the early stages, is more likely to be successful in engaging men and developing the trust needed to facilitate verbal communication.

Notes

1. 'Intimate' is used here and throughout this chapter to indicate a long-term, sexual partnership and whilst recognising that such terms are highly contested they seem adequately clear to serve an heuristic purpose.
2. The same point clearly holds true for sexually transmitted diseases in heterosexual relationships and, as Lorber and Moore (2002: 129) point out, this leaves gay men in the same position now that heterosexual women have always been where penetrative sex represents both risk and trust.

5   Men engaging with health care

Introduction

It has become almost taken for granted in health professional literature that men delay seeking help for health concerns and access primary care services (usually meaning GP practices) less frequently than women (see, for example, Banks 2001; Griffiths 2001; Holroyd 2002; Lloyd 2001). Explanations for this delay and difference in consultation rates vary but are usually predicated on stereotypes of women's greater compliance and higher morbidity and men's stoicism and reluctance to ask for help, which together are said to explain the 'women get sicker, but men die quicker' health patterns in the UK. However, research carried out at the MRC Social and Public Health Sciences Unit in Glasgow (reviewed in Chapter 2) has raised questions about such generalizations regarding sex differences in both morbidity reporting (Macintyre et al. 1996; Macintyre et al. 1999) and GP attendance (Hunt et al. 1999). Together these publications suggest that reporting and attendance are determined primarily by severity of symptoms or specific condition type and that there is no statistical evidence for a generalized excess morbidity reporting or GP attendance among women. The exception being for psychological distress/mental health where there is a consistent pattern of higher rates of female reporting (Macintyre et al. 1996) and GP attendance (Hunt et al. 1999).

Other recent research by Seymour-Smith et al. (2002) has used discourse analysis to explore how health professionals working in primary care in the UK construct masculinity, make sense of their male patients, and the possible implications of this for health promotion work with men. This work identifies how hegemonic masculine traits were both criticized, for their potentially detrimental effects on health, yet also 'valorized and indulged' by the health professionals. This work does more than identify the stereotypes that the health professionals hold, it shows how these representations become frameworks for action that can create or restrict opportunities within the surgery setting for 'what is possible and what various potential performances of masculinity might mean and how they might be interpreted' (Seymour-Smith et al. 2002: 265). In this respect, as Robertson (1998) has previously highlighted, the way health professionals understand masculinity may be just as significant as how lay men understand it for facilitating or restricting men's access to primary care services. This may particularly be the case for those men not holding to hegemonic masculine values.

This chapter responds to the exhortations in the MRC Social and Public Health Sciences Unit research papers cited above to pay attention to the social context of gendered help-seeking behaviour. It also expands on the work of Seymour-Smith et al. (2002) by heeding their statement that future research should consider how masculine identities, particularly marginalized or subordinated masculinities, are negotiated in the process of becoming (or indeed not becoming) a 'male patient' in primary care settings. The first section builds on the arguments initiated in Chapter 2 by looking further at how responsibility for health is constructed. The second section looks more specifically at how this impacts on the processes of engaging with services. An argument is made that simplistic assertions of male stoicism and delay in accessing services cannot be sustained consistently and that utilisation (or not) of primary care services is integrally tied into gendered identity and specifically the demarcation made between 'health', which is not related to GPs and health services, and 'illness', which is.

The politics of responsibility

As discussed in Chapter 2, it is often asserted in both the media (for example, Stepney 1996; Lyons and Willott 1999; Hammond 2000) and health professional literature (for example, Griffiths 1999; Banks 2001) that men do not take responsibility for their health and that their behaviour (usually termed 'risk taking') also shows an inherently irresponsible approach to health and well-being. Here I look at how responsibility for 'men's health' is constructed by the men and the health professionals in this study and link this to wider debates about individual versus collective and authoritative versus negotiated approaches to health promotion (Beattie 1991).

(Ir)responsible lifestyles

Despite a general concurrence with the view that men were not 'health conscious', all the men indicated that, as individuals, they had a responsibility for their own health in terms of lifestyle choices. As Ron makes clear: 'I mean, if you wanna change something in your life there's only *you* can do it. If you wanna stop smoking *you've* gotta stop smoking. If you wanna stop eating bloody fatty foods its *you* who's got to stop eating fatty foods' (Ron, DM3).

This was frequently tied into narratives about issues of control, independence and a specifically hegemonic masculine rejection of authoritative intervention regarding lifestyle choices that has been noted in previous research (Sharpe and Arnold 1999) on men, health and lifestyle:

SR: You mentioned smoking and stuff earlier, do you think with those sorts of lifestyle things that blokes feel less pressure to comply than women?

Hugh: I just think blokes will do it when they want to do it. They won't be told. Its like anyone could tell me I need to stop smoking but I'll do it when I'm ready to stop smoking and not when someone tells me to [. . .] I think I'd listen to a doctor. I watch all the adverts and I do think, yeah, I should stop smoking and that. But I'm not ready to stop smoking, you know I might never be ready to stop. If a doctor tells me 'You need to stop smoking' then it's my decision whether I do or don't.

(Hugh, CABS2)

Many narratives reflected this idea of negotiated power when considering responsibility for health. There was a general feeling that health professionals, and doctors in particular, hold specialist knowledge and that a degree of trust in them is required (see also Lupton 1996) but that this should not entail a wholesale relinquishing of individual responsibility or control:

Dan: I leave my trust in them [health services], not completely, but I expect them to help and support communities, and people who work, everybody. You can't always know everything, so they need to keep informing us of what's good, what's bad, what's indifferent [. . .] Ultimately its like anything, you can be told numerous amounts of things, but you can't force folk. We all know, for example, smoking's bad for us and I'm sure the NHS has promoted that a thousand times or more. We know that, but we don't do anything, generally very few of us do actually adhere to it and actually go to their guidelines and follow it right through. But it does need to be in place.

(Dan, CABS7)

Bloor and McIntosh (1990) suggest from their empirical work that the apparent power/knowledge discrepancy present in lay–professional interactions is what actually creates space for resistance. I would further suggest that such resistance itself is often gendered in its demonstration. Whereas women's resistance may be an active, but often hidden, ignoring of advice, such as that found between mothers and health visitors (Bloor and McIntosh 1990), accounts here suggest that men frequently and publicly use (rhetorical and/or actual) resistance to health advice as a way of demonstrating masculinity. As outlined in Chapter 2, such resistance can form part of the 'don't care' rhetoric necessary to suggest conformation to hegemonic masculine values:

SR: I'm just wondering if you think that how men think about health is different to how women think about it?

Quinn: Yeah, cause it's important to women innit but blokes don't really bother about it. I mean speaking from my experience, like I say I never think about it.

(Quinn, DM2)

This explicit (masculine) desire to retain control and reject interference in everyday lifestyle choices ('being told what to do' – Sharpe and Arnold 1999) conflicts with the aim of 'surveillance medicine' (Armstrong 1983, 1995) to extend the boundaries of medical dominion and control over those currently 'healthy' as well as those unwell. Armstrong (1995) suggests that the rise of this new surveillance medicine from the beginning of the twentieth century relies on dissolving previous distinctions between 'health' and 'illness', thus postulating all as being potentially 'at risk' in terms of their health and well-being, through what he terms a 'problematization of the normal' (Armstrong 1995: 395). Yet a health/illness distinction was clearly maintained by most of the men, many of who continue to see health as a 'normal/natural' state (see Chapter 2). In this sense, the power of surveillance medicine to extend dominion and control is diluted by men's gendered reticence to conform and accept such authoritative control. It was apparent that 'lifestyle messages' did become internalized by the men as all listed similar 'behaviours' as key to reducing health risks (for example, exercise, low-fat diets) or increasing health risks (for example, excess alcohol, smoking, fatty foods). Yet this internalization may do little to influence practices that are embedded in larger social contexts. When the 'risk' discourse of health promotion messages conflict with (hegemonic) male discourses of autonomy, independence, and the pragmatic requirements of men's everyday lives, it is often found wanting in its ability to influence men's health-related practices.

Whilst reinforcing ideas of individual autonomy and responsibility for health, the narratives of the gay men were some of the few that also indicated that individual lifestyle choices can have collective consequences. This was paramount in narratives about sexual practices and was so prominent an issue for all of the gay men that it was often bound into their definitions of health:

SR: I was hoping that you might give me some of your ideas on what health is . . .

David: Health is the welfare of yourself, the welfare of people around you, in the sense of . . . especially for a gay man, if you're having safe sex that's obviously a big health issue. If you're not having safe sex, then you're risking your health and you're risking other people's health – if you don't know who they've been with and they don't know who

> you've been with – to get a sexually transmitted disease or even HIV
> and AIDS.
>
> (David, GM1)

Heterosexual men were frequently castigated in these narratives for their ignorance and selfish, irresponsible sexual ('health') practices that put others at risk, as were some promiscuous gay men, particularly those known to be HIV positive:

> I know of one person, I've known he's HIV for the last six years and I'm only one of three or four people that know he's HIV. Yet he's very active on the gay scene, and I've actually brought this up in conversation with one or two people at [HIV/AIDS charity]. I said, 'I know full damn well this guy's going out there screwing around and he's putting, not only himself, but he's putting other people at risk' but there's not much you can do except educate people.
>
> (Wayne, GM6)

For the gay men in this age group the risk rhetoric of HIV/AIDS was far from abstract. As mentioned earlier, and highlighted in previous research (Hart et al. 1990), many of these men had lost close friends and partners through the late 1980s, early 1990s, and narratives about the need for self-surveillance, part of the process of extending disciplinary power in surveillance medicine (Nettleton 1995: 113ff), were reinforced through real accounts and experiences of confronting death. In such circumstances, 'lifestyle choices' can shift from being part of an unconscious 'logic of practice' (Bourdieu 1990; Williams 1995), to being conscious decisions. This is not to say that choices become robotlike, predetermined by powerful ('risk') discourses and personal experiences, rather, consciousness enters into and becomes an additional player in exerting influence on (health) practices. By the time of the second interview, David had engaged in (what in his terms was) unsafe sex with a new partner. Despite a strong commitment to 'safe sex' as part of individual and collective responsibility for health, David's need to develop emotional capital, as part of the process of giving and receiving affection and expressing trust in a new relationship, became more pressing. It is in this way that 'habitus' (Bourdieu 1977) can become unstable as previously acquired sets of generative dispositions become challenged by the incorporation of new experiences, consciousness, and the role of action-orientated embodied emotionality as outlined in Chapter 4.

Health professionals, lifestyles and responsibility

This experience of men not responding to, or overtly resenting, 'lifestyle' change advice was common to all the health professionals. Three went further in agreeing with the opinion above that health is a 'normal/natural' state and that 'lifestyle' choices should not require health professional intervention:

> I think it's right that we should assume wellness. I think a healthy society assumes wellness. I think someone between 25–35 years who doesn't assume they're healthy for whatever reason has actually got a bit of a problem. I think you're in the peak of everything aren't you. To not assume that, to not make assumptions about your own good state of health and physical well-being, is a bit sad really and I think most men do that and rightly so.
>
> (Collette, HP2)

> At the end of the day I see it as there are a lot of do-gooders wandering around trying to change people's health who don't actually want it bloody changing. They're just jumping to different tunes from the government.
>
> (Ian, HP4)

In this respect, although the move towards the 'problematization of the normal', identified through a focus on 'lifestyle choices' in health promotion, may be a discourse presently enshrined in UK health policy, it is clear that not all community health professionals see health promotion in this way (Adams et al. 2002). As others have noted (Nettleton and Bunton 1995: 57), there has been little research examining the 'perceptions, activities and knowledge base [of those] concerned with the delivery of health promotion programmes'. And accounts here question the assumption, often inherently present though not overtly stated in health surveillance critiques of health promotion, which postulates all health professionals as passive, willing and unquestioning participants in the rise of 'medicalisation' and surveillance medicine culture.

Even for those health professionals committed to the importance of promoting specific lifestyle choices there was a general feeling or recognition that giving such advice was often ineffective:

> Interestingly in the early 90s, when we were looking at this [well-men clinics], we were trying to give men information about the importance of not smoking, healthy lifestyle, cutting down on

alcohol, and I felt that you could tell them till you were blue in the face but they didn't believe you.

(Adam, HP1)

Either you're motivated, you come to the doctor and you're that type of person you're going to stick to it, or you're not. Opportunistic health promotion, to me, doesn't seem to have achieved much. I know research says that it does, but I honestly don't think I've ever successfully managed to get anyone to stop smoking for instance.

(Fiona, CP7)

For many of the health professionals this ineffectiveness was seen to be part of a larger, structural issue relating to inequalities in class, income, education, that therefore took the responsibility for men's health out of the health service to wider social policy considerations:

SR: Do you think that those sorts of inequality issues are particularly important around men's health?

Collette: Well I don't think we are born on a level playing field. I think the day a child comes into the world there's inequality and I don't think it's just in health, it affects where they go into school, it affects how they access services, it affects their ability to relate to those things and their education and it's just incredibly unfair. I think as health visitors we're very aware of that unfairness. I don't know how we address it, I don't know cause I think addressing it has to come from central government.

(Collette, HP2)

Yet such narratives were rare and it was more common for emphasis to be placed on the intractability of men's behaviour and their reluctance to comply with lifestyle advice. Whilst such narratives about the (in)effectiveness of lifestyle advice were not always directed solely at men, they were generally associated with, or juxtaposed to, narratives about women's greater compliance to such advice, this in turn being linked to their reproductive role and/or their greater involvement with GP services from a young age:

I think women certainly have a far more well-developed sense of preventive health care than men ever will do. But women are brought up to realize that they need to have regular cervical smearing and they are used to going to the doctor for problems which aren't directly related to ill-health.

(John, CP3)

> Men of that age [25–40 years] tend not to access the services, or don't have a great deal of contact with primary care in general. Women tend to have more access because that age tends to be child-bearing age, so they have contact with midwives, health visitors, they bring the children into surgery, and they also have the on-going cervical cytology programme. So they tend to have a lot more contact.
>
> (Dawn, CP5)

Such narratives become part of a wider discourse that, as feminist writers and researchers have shown, continues the medicalization, surveillance, and thereby control of female bodies (Petersen and Lupton 1996: 72*ff*). Yet the construction of the female body as 'other', that postulates it as a subject for the (male) medical gaze, also has the concomitant effect of obscuring the male body that represents the 'norm' and thereby becomes taken for granted. This in turn can create a situation where men are likely to be ignored or overlooked by health service providers (Buchbinder 1998: 358), and this issue will be addressed further in the second section.

Rolling back the state: what of the NHS?

This medicalization of everyday life and the rise of surveillance medicine is bound to the social policy context in which it occurs. The shift towards individual responsibility for health sits well with wider neoliberal policy moves in the UK to withdraw state responsibility for key areas of welfare since the 1970s (Petersen and Lupton 1996: 174*ff*; Baggot 2000: 248). 'Individualization' has become a cornerstone of the revisioned notions of citizenship, conceived by Conservative governments through the late 1980s and early 1990s and continued under the current Labour government (Higgs 1998: 186*ff*) and it is of interest that the rise of the term 'health promotion', and associated notions of risk, have coincided with this shift from collectivism to liberalism in UK social policy (Farrant 1991; Parish 1995). It was clear that such policy ideas had directly influenced a minority of the men with two suggesting that reducing NHS provision for services, making health provision cost money, would improve individual lifestyle choices, as Kiaran points out:

> If I'm talking about the National Health Service now, I sometimes wonder if it does more harm than good. If we all had to take responsibility for our own health instead of just thinking 'Well they'll sort us out.' If I think 'Well I smoke, I'll get cancer, they'll treat it, and it won't cost me anything'. But if I thought 'If I get cancer I'll have to pay out all this money to get it treated', I might

think twice. It's a different way of looking at health in general; you keep yourself healthier if you've got to pay out.

(Kiaran, GM4)

This was a minority view, though. Linked to the distinction outlined earlier that the men made between health and illness, it was also common to make a distinction between the role the NHS has in treating those who are unwell and its potential role in helping people to keep well or stay well. Some men felt that the NHS had little to offer those already 'well':

I think it's [NHS] got a responsibility to get you well, but it doesn't have a responsibility to keep you well, that's down to yourself.'

(Frank, DM6)

I don't feel that the NHS should have to help me out to keep myself healthy and balanced. I'm an individual and if I am wanting to keep myself healthy and keep myself active then I know what I want.

(Peter, DM1)

SR: Do you think that the National Health Service has a responsibility in helping you to stay well?

QUINN: No. No, I think it should be like it is. You know if you injure yourself then you go and get sorted, but it's not down to them to make sure you're all right in everyday life. It's down to you innit.

(Quinn, DM2)

It is perhaps no coincidence that these narratives, rejecting input from the NHS in staying well, were most commonly and strongly expressed by the disabled men and those men with chronic illnesses. As stated in earlier chapters, and highlighted in the work of Williams (1993) and Galvin (2002), a significant part of presenting oneself as a 'morally good' citizen when chronically ill or impaired is to sustain the highest amount of independence possible. When these discourses coalesce with discourses of (hegemonic) male autonomy, such narratives become a means of sustaining a virtuous (male) identity.

For the majority of men, and health professionals, there was general agreement that health services should be active in providing clear, up-to-date health information that was well distributed using marketing techniques and the support of the media (this is discussed further in the second section). This approach tended to represent a conflation of health promotion with health education, the provision of health information (Tones 1997), and implies to an extent that there was little that could, or even should, be done by health services beyond this 'awareness raising'. Such conflation was not only found in the interviews with the men but was also present at times in the interviews with health professionals, as the following implies:

> Men of that age group are exposed to health promotion but probably don't respond to that. I think when you are seeing people of that age group for opportunistic illnesses, which is usually when you do see them, or injuries, and you happen to try and do a bit of ongoing health promotion, they are aware of the issues around how much they should be drinking, they shouldn't be smoking, what their diet ought to be, but its not ranked as something that's particularly important to them.
>
> (John, HP3)

Screening men out?

A small number of men also felt that the NHS should have a role in the provision of 'screening' services for men. This tended to be tied in with their narratives about the physiological body (see Chapter 3) and a belief that pathological changes could take place, unrecognized by the experiential body, that could be detected by health professionals performing 'checks' and this could lead to early intervention and better health outcomes:

> But they've [NHS] just got to keep making men more aware, even if it means bombarding them every six months with men's health checks and things like that. I went for mine. I can't even remember when it was but it's while I've been married, and it was just normal stuff, blood pressure and if it's high for 20 years then you've got a problem but if it's high when you're in your 20s they can sort it out.
>
> (Owen, CABS5)

However, these narratives often oscillated with other narratives about how such services would be seen by the majority of men; as Owen goes on to explain:

> But perhaps men won't go, they need ... if its voluntary to go and have your men's health check then perhaps a high proportion of men won't go [...] If they did regular health checks then the response rate wouldn't be high, you know, because it's the ignorance and they don't want to change, men.
>
> (Owen, CABS5)

Here Owen uses health as a way of representing himself as a morally good citizen, pursuing the 'should care' discourse (see Chapter 2), despite the fact that this risks having his male identity ridiculed. This could also be, as

Wetherell and Edley (1999) point out, because it has almost become the 'new hegemony' to show public rejection of (previously?) hegemonic aspects of masculinity in late modernity, and this in itself represents a further form of 'doing' hegemonic masculinity, demonstrating one's independent thought, autonomy and thereby being one's 'own man'.

For the gay men 'screening', usually meaning regular checks for sexually transmitted diseases, was very much part of acculturation into the gay 'life-style' (Flowers et al. 1998).

> *Kiaran:* I think gay men it's slightly different, they would look after them-selves, they probably would go more [to health services]. Like a lot of gay men will go to the GUM Clinic for sexual health reasons. I don't know whether straight men do the same unless they've had some-thing and they've had to and then they carry on going after that. But to go in for regular checks...
>
> *SR:* So the GUM Clinic is quite an acceptable place for gay men to go for regular screening?
>
> *Kiaran:* Yeah, I think it is, yeah.
>
> *SR:* How does that process of familiarity start do you think for most gay men?
>
> *Kiaran:* I suppose they usually go because they get a partner that goes regularly and find out about it, they hear about it. Yeah, and nobody is like ashamed to say 'Oh I went to the GUM clinic last week' you know what I mean. People will say it.
>
> (Kiaran, GM4)

It was therefore seen as a duty of the NHS to provide such services *and* for individual gay men to use them. Doing so represents a form of shared knowledge/experience, differentiates from that which is 'straight', and thus contributes to a common, shared, 'gay' identity.

Narratives about screening and health promotion services were often tied to narratives about the fiscal crisis and limited resources within the NHS. In this way, many of the men positioned health promotion services very much as an 'added extra' that could be provided once the NHS had met its (more important) 'illness' commitments:

> *SR:* Do you think the National Health Service should have a role in helping men stay well?
>
> *Bob:* In the maintenance respect, yes, fantastic as another part to the service yes, because it's a fabulous service it really is. It's virtually free, I mean National Insurance is pence, you're not paying into anything really. As another part of it yeah, I mean if there are the resources there to do it, without affecting current standards then yeah. But are

they not stretched a little bit far at the moment, I would have thought so.

(Bob, CABS6)

The health professionals recognized this perception of the NHS as being a 'disease service' (John, HP3) and in addition were not always convinced that 'well men' represented an appropriate client group when they were already exceptionally busy caring for those with acute or chronic illness:

Well it's not our main ... certainly from my kind of background [practice nurse], the main purpose is to deal with the client group you've got, sort of shoved in your face [laugh] because you've got a busy caseload. You are aware of issues surrounding your males, but trying to get round to sort of being pro-active in that area is quite difficult.

(Dawn, HP5)

Previous empirical work has also shown that 'well men' are not prioritized as a client group by community health professionals (Williams 1997) or in strategic health service plans (MORI 1995), particularly when resources are scarce. When men's and health professionals' narratives about scarce resources coincide with the idea that (for men) 'health' is a normal/natural state, it becomes clear why surveillance of those (men) presently 'healthy' is not a priority for a service struggling to meet its commitments to treating those currently unwell.

In concluding this section, the narrow focus (by both the men and the health professionals) on the role that health services have in raising awareness of health issues reflects the way that health promotion is often conflated to health education when implemented within a neoliberal health policy environment. Yet the shifting of responsibility for health back to the individual within this policy context is not a gender-neutral process and this focus (on awareness raising) allows men to maintain autonomy and avoid what can be seen as medical interference in everyday life. It creates opportunities for men to demonstrate both a 'don't care' discourse (by rejecting health advice) and a 'should care' discourse (by claiming themselves as independently responsible for their health) which, as previous chapters and the following section highlight, are mobilized in different ways and at different times to (re)construct masculine identity/identities. Screening services create a particular point of conflict for some of those interviewed as they require a degree of submission of autonomy and clash with narratives of health as a 'normal/natural' state for men. When health services are seen as (only) being responsible for those currently unwell, 'well-men' services can come to represent an oxymoron for some men (and health professionals).

Towards marriage or war? Processes of engagement

Having considered how responsibility for health is constructed, this section looks specifically at how these constructions are negotiated in different ways and at different times to facilitate or limit men's access to primary care services. It continues to link this to wider debates within health promotion.

Being well (and) informed

As shown in the previous section, issues of providing health information seem paramount when thinking about what constituted engaging with 'health promotion' both for men and health professionals. The specific targeting of health information for men was something that many felt was currently not done well enough, particularly in comparison to the amount of information available to women:

> You can ask any man, gay, straight, they'd probably say, in health, there's more publicity, leaflets, flyers and advertising aimed at females and their health, than male. For example, pregnancy, taking the pill, breast cancer and things like that. I think there's a lot more literature for the females than the guys out there.
>
> (David, GM1)

> If you look at the media, newspapers and magazines, it tends to be more information about women having screening programmes. You occasionally see articles about the importance of testicular self-examination, prostatic problems in men, but I would suggest that they are less pressured ... they don't tend to see as much, as many articles promoting that sort of health screening.
>
> (Adam, HP1)

This perceived inequity of information helps create and sustain the idea of health as a female 'field' or domain. Yet, as Adam implies, and Lyons and Willott (1999) point out, such a gender focus may also be beneficial to men in relieving them of the 'pressure' of having to think about or act on such information and advice and this is considered further later.

Significant importance was given by a number of men and health professionals to the potential role of the media in helping raise awareness of health-related issues and thereby alter men's health-related practices. This was felt to be best achieved through the inclusion of health advice, well-man checks, and signs/symptoms of specific diseases (testicular cancer and prostate diseases being most commonly mentioned) on television, particularly in soap operas:

> I still think the likes of [health] issues in Coronation Street, East-
> enders, even reading it in the newspaper, is the only way you're
> gonna change men's attitudes.
>
> (Martin, CABS3)

> People will believe what comes out of the little box in the corner of
> the living room. I actually wrote to the producers of Coronation St
> and asked them to ... spoke about why don't they get someone like
> Jack Duckworth to go to his doctors for a well-man check; tell him he
> smokes too much, tell him he drinks too much, tell him he eats the
> wrong foods.
>
> (Adam, HP1)

Such approaches were also seen by the health professionals to be a particularly effective way of targeting messages to men often termed 'hard to
reach', seen to have unhealthy lifestyles, and therefore generally poorer
health outcomes, as Adam goes on to explain:

> As a health professional it's very frustrating to try and give good
> advice, correct advice, knowing full well it goes in one ear and out
> the other. But people of lower socio-economic groups will more
> readily accept the tabloid newspaper or stuff coming out of the TV.
>
> (Adam, HP1)

Yet for other health professionals raising awareness of potential health
problems was also seen as being (potentially) iatrogenic, having the effect of
increasing the number of 'worried well' seeking help:

> The promotion of the testicular cancer certainly has generated quite
> a lot of interest and maybe more neurotic and anxious people will
> come in [laugh] [...] Locally, that was an issue because [local per-
> sonality] had testicular cancer and generated quite a lot of awareness
> amongst younger people. It might be a bit mean to say this, but I
> think it tends to be in those who are a little over anxious anyway and
> I'm sure I've not picked up any pathology out of the extra increase in
> people that I've seen.
>
> (John, HP3)

A difference was sustained here by these health professionals between
lifestyle advice, which is acceptable to impart but not enforce, and potential
pathological changes, where imparting knowledge merely creates anxiety.
This was quite often the antithesis of what men wanted from engagement
with health education and information, which was not to be told how to live

their lives but to have adequate information about when to recognize that physiological processes were breaking down.

Shifting male culture

The issue of information, and the links between this and changing men's lifestyle choices, was often seen to be a question of altering specific aspects of (male) culture and tradition. To this extent, it was commonplace to raise the importance of the education system and habits developed early in life as one (and possibly the only) way to change men's reluctance to engage with health advice and health services. This was seen to be important in two different but related ways; first, in getting health education messages across when men (as boys) would be most receptive:

> A lot of that can, and should, be done within the school, that's where they can get the information across. [...] Once you put that information in, they may never use it, but it's there if they want to and, at the end of the day, people are free to make their own choices.
>
> (Collette, HP2)

Second, this could facilitate a change of culture and a challenging of (hegemonic) male stereotypes, particularly those about men being uninterested in health, through schools or when young:

> SR: I'm keen to think about how health promotion services might be made more acceptable and accessible to men.
>
> Tony: It's a difficult one. I suppose it all comes down to health education in schools. That's a key issue, a key time to bring it in through the education system because that's where people get the stereotypes, the 'macho' ideal thing from.
>
> (Tony, DM5)

> The problem in getting men ... it's got to start in schools, it's got to be part of their kind of education and their sort of whole culture, their attitude towards what health is [...] they've got to change their culture, their attitude to accept that accessing health promotion activities is normal and is important.
>
> (Dawn, HP5)

The narratives here are specifically those of 'normalization'. What is being suggested is that the process of seeking help and caring for health can be instilled as 'normal', acceptable, behaviour for men during the early years thus increasing contact with health services even when well. As Nettleton

(1995: 113*ff*) highlights, Foucault's (1979) discussion of disciplinary power, which she and others have suggested maps onto 'surveillance medicine', relies on three main instruments:

- *hierarchical observation* referring to the sites where people can be observed, schools being one such site;
- *normalizing judgement* where actions and attributes of individuals are compared to others thus allowing a norm or standard to be developed; and
- *the examination*, which combines the first two and creates a situation where individuals can be assessed and if necessary corrected.

Yet, as pointed out in the previous section, the rise of surveillance medicine is not devoid of gendered social context. Whilst the narratives of both the men and health professionals suggest that the above instruments of disciplinary power would need to be brought to bear if surveillance medicine was to extend to men, they also recognized that this would require a large cultural shift. To put it in Bourdieu's (1977, 1990) terms, men would need to acquire a different set of generative dispositions (*habitus*), thus altering the current logic of their (health) practices. Thinking about this further, under patriarchy, hegemonic masculinity becomes bound into health service structures and it is a (hegemonic) male gaze that undertakes observation and examination and a (hegemonic) male 'norm' by which others (women, non-hegemonic men) are measured (White 2002: 131).[1] In this way, as those wielding the tools and being at the top of a gendered 'hierarchy', it is unlikely that (hegemonic) men themselves would, or could, become the subject of such instruments of disciplinary power and thus acquire this changed set of generative dispositions (see also Rosenfeld and Faircloth 2006).

A small detour is necessary here to elucidate this point. When considering the historical development of health services, great emphasis has been placed on how the poor health status of male recruits during the Boer War acted as one of the driving forces behind the later development of the welfare state within the UK (Fraser 1984). Yet the (male-led) development of health promotion/education services around this time did very little directly to target information or health promotion campaigns towards such men. Rather, as Welshman's (1997) work on health education during this period shows, such services and campaigns were more often targeted at mothers, infants and schoolchildren. The sites of hierarchical observation, where normalizing judgements were made and examinations undertaken, were, and still are, rarely those that adult men frequent.[2] As feminists have rightly pointed out, it was the poor state of *men's* health that generated cause for concern. Yet, the patriarchal nature of health service structures determined that subsequent actions – including the development of a health visiting service, the establishment of maternal and infant welfare clinics, and an expansion of school health services – focused attention (and thereby responsibility) specifically on women and children. As Welshman (1997: 204) highlights 'women were regarded as the guardians of family health'. Consideration of men's (health) needs may have prompted action, but the gendered, patriarchal nature of health and wider social structures leads to a situation where men can remain obfuscated as the beneficiaries of subsequent service development.

Avoiding the 'gaze'

As shown above, such obfuscation of men from surveillance and the medical gaze is not abstract and often occurs through the reinforcement of hegemonic masculine ideals in daily life. For many of the men this was related to (hegemonic) notions of male strength and independence with frequent and powerful narratives that presented men as being the serious users of the health service (see also Seymour-Smith et al. 2002):

> No, no, I don't go to the doctor unless I'm desperate. I think I've been once in 6 or 7 years . . . If there's something really bad with me then I would go, I wouldn't be scared of going [. . .] But I don't go running to the doctors [. . .] I look at it, the less I go to the doctors, the better off everyone else is that's poorly. You know, I'm not taking his time up.
>
> (Hugh, CABS2)

Such narratives were echoed by the health professionals although these were always linked to the potentially detrimental effects of holding to such notions: 'Anecdotally, I think men are poor at accessing health preventive services, more likely to put up with a problem. Put up with it, put up with it, until it might be too late in the case of something like testicular cancer' (Adam, HP1).

As Adam suggests, such representations rely on the juxtaposition of the sexes, this being built upon supposed 'natural' and 'common sense' differences between men and women, as Hugh goes on to explain:

> They always say women are hypochondriacs don't they? I know me mum is, she's never away from the doctors and there's always summit wrong with her. Where to me I just, I'll get over it myself, unless I'm in a lot of pain or can't shift it or whatever, then I'll go and see him.
>
> (Hugh, CABS2)

In addition, as Connell (1995) points out, hegemonic masculinity is also constructed, often unconsciously, as being thoroughly heterosexual, and the haptic experience associated with health screening can carry an implicit suggestion of potentially homosexual (and therefore to be rejected) activity as the following narrative highlights:

> *SR:* Would there be any advantage in setting up similar [screening] programmes for men?
>
> *Martin:* Absolutely, but you'd struggle to get the men there. I think men like to feel secure in their own health and certainly they don't want to find anything wrong with them. I guess they don't want to be embarrassed like ... [SR: Embarrassed?] Yeah, stood in the middle of surgery and says 'Right drop your trousers'. I don't think any man wants that. Whereas women they've always been led, like smear tests, they've always been told they've got to get it done, it's in their own interest and they've come round to it. Whereas men don't want to be 'right drop your trousers, cough', they don't want it.
>
> (Martin, CABS3)

For those men who specifically constructed identities in contrast to hegemonic masculinity, compliance with screening, surveillance and familiarity with health services can become 'normalized' as shown in the discussion of gay men and sexual health screening in the previous section. This is not to say that access to services for these men was unproblematic as we shall see shortly.

Such obfuscation of (some) men of health surveillance services and processes represents a double-edged sword and creates a clear tension within the men's narratives. This was often visible in men's insistence that they should have the same right to health information and screening services as women but that 'most men' (not usually the man talking!) would not utilize such services. Whilst allowing the (clearly desired) non-intervention of medical services into aspects of daily life, this obfuscation also created the potential risk that early detrimental changes to physiological processes could go unrecognized, which could then cause longer term problems.

Legitimating engagement

Having established the specific ways that hegemonic masculine discourses were mobilized to avoid medical intervention it is also important to establish what narratives men mobilize to legitimate engagement with services. It is via processes of legitimization that men can mediate and manage the 'don't care, should care' dichotomy outlined in Chapter 2. The distinction between health and illness maintained by the men not only serves to preclude health professional involvement in daily life but also ensures that access to services *is* legitimated when they are in a state of ill health. Having a clearly identifiable illness, or particularly injury, was seen by all the men as valid reason for attending health services, although this was often further justified by reiterating that it would have to be serious:

> *SR:* You don't have any particular problems or qualms about phoning up the doctors to make an appointment?
>
> *Martin:* No. I haven't got no qualms with going to see a doctor at all.
>
> *SR:* So a lot of this stuff about men delaying going . . .
>
> *Martin:* Oh men do delay. I delay, but it doesn't bother me going to see a doctor, but you just don't think 'I'm gonna see a doctor'. You think, 'Well it's not really that bad I'll see how it is in a couple of weeks.'
>
> (Martin, CABS3)

Legitimate engagement with health services was also achieved when the health/illness distinction was destabilized or disrupted in some way. Both the men and the health professionals recognized the importance and impact of ill health in someone close as one of the few triggers that allowed men to initiate contact with health services even if currently well:

> As you get older you tend to think about it [health] a bit more. Plus your parents are getting older, you start losing older relatives, and mortality starts to creep into the agenda!
>
> (Kiaran, GM4)

> The men I come across it's in a well-man clinic, and usually as a result of a relative, or perhaps a friend, that's recently died. It could be a relative that's had a heart attack, it could be a friend that's had something like testicular cancer. It triggers something in their mind that they ought to get checked out.
>
> (Adam, HP1)

Again, these narratives draw on real or observed experiences that elucidate physiological processes as vulnerable and it is recognition of this vulnerability that can (legitimately) trigger engagement with primary care services. Clearly linked into these narratives is the significance of family histories in decisions about whether something may require health professional attention and this is highlighted vividly in Martin's narrative:

> My father died of skin cancer when I was very young. So, if I've got a scratch on me back I think 'Is that a mole?', I always get me mum to check that out, she says, 'Right you ought to go and see a doctor'.

So certain things like that I'm very cautious about. I always run it by them.

(Martin, CABS3)

In this regard, as previous research has shown (Hunt et al. 2000a, 2000b), family history can have a significant impact on the construction of lay health beliefs and practices with this again being mediated through notions of risk, vulnerability and physiological embodiment.

A further area highlighted by Martin's quote, and present in other men's narratives, is the importance for men of 'significant others' in legitimating engagement with services. Many examples were provided by the men of female partners, or mothers, taking responsibility for either encouraging or directly making health service appointments, and this was echoed in the experience of the health professionals:

SR: So if you were worried about something that didn't seem to be going away would you make the appointment?

Hugh: Jane sorts things like that. I've always had me life sorted out you see with being in the army, you know everything's been done for me. Before I met Jane me mum used to sort everything out for me, Jane does now. If I need to be there, tell me when I have to be there and I'll be there. But when it comes to me making the appointments I'm not very good at that kind of thing.

(Hugh, CABS2)

A lot of blokes still need their mummies. And this is where wives come in. They're surrogate mothers a lot of women aren't they. They need to be looked after, men. Left to our own devices we don't look after ourselves. I think it takes a woman behind the bulk of blokes to actually get them to look after themselves. It takes that woman's nagging.

(Ian, HP4)

The targeting of female partners as a means of getting health promotion messages across to men was a common suggestion, and actual practice amongst the health professionals. However, as indicated by the regular use of the term 'nagging' in these narratives, it was also perceived as being potentially disruptive to intimate, 'pure' relationships that Giddens (1992) claims are premised on mutual respect and emotional democracy, not reliance, in late modernity. These narratives, combined with those discussed in previous chapters of female partners helping men to 'settle down' into healthier lifestyles, and general narratives of women caring more about health and well-being, create and sustain discourses that collectively can be recognized as the 'feminization of health'. This feminization of health does not necessarily extend to illness and this is reflected in the division of labour in primary care services where health promotion and screening services are predominantly delivered by female staff (practice nurses, health visitors, female GPs) and more prestigious illness services by male staff (GPs).

Health work, places and spaces

Such feminization of health did not remain at the level of the abstract but had direct and identifiable consequences in relation to access of services. General practitioner practices, in particular, were seen as female gendered space, although they were a legitimate (though not necessarily comfortable) space for men when unwell:

> Women are more used to going to the GP from a younger age, puberty, periods and then pregnancy, all this sort of thing. Whereas men, well the only time we ever go is with your mum and dad if you've got a cold, or measles, and then maybe if you've got a bit of an injury or flu or something later on.
>
> (Francis, CABS1)

> Using the service isn't the most attractive or appealing thing to me and I would imagine to most men similar to me. The fact that you go and sit in a waiting room with kids, grandmas, coughing people, and it's hot and stuffy, and there's a magazine, *Woman's Own*, *Country Life*, on the table and you've got some pain in your chest or something. And I don't really wanna go, but you're forced to go because you know there is something wrong with you. And just actually the process of going to the doctor's, and being checked, and waiting, it's an ordeal really. *And there's not many people in there you can relate to.*
>
> (Dan, CABS7, emphasis added)

This same situation was recognized in the health professionals' narratives:

> Well you don't tend to see men apart from in a sort of emergency-type situation, or you see the older men because they're ill. Whereas women are coming in all the time for the pill or for the babies or whatever.
>
> (Fiona, HP7)

Recognition of this gendering of GP surgeries, and the concomitant difficulty of not accessing men in their middle years, led to discussions about undertaking health work with men in alternative settings. Many of the men and health professionals were already aware, through the media or health professional literature, that such work, taking health services to where men congregate, was already being carried out in various settings.

Pubs and clubs represented a male gendered space that was raised in these discussions although views varied regarding the appropriateness and effectiveness of this setting. Whilst three men felt that this would be an appropriate setting for health promotion work with men (usually discussed in terms of the provision of health-related information), the other three men and one health professional who commented felt it would be an unwelcome intrusion and imposition into men's social activity that would therefore prove ineffective:

> I've tried to speak to people about health, in a night club, give out leaflets and things. It doesn't work because they're with their mates, out having a few beers and it's a social night, so it's the wrong place to try and bring this health promotion message across because it's a social night they're having.
>
> (David, GM1)

> I've spoken to health visitors who've said we should go out sit in pubs and do health education there. But I think there's got to be a commitment by the person wanting the health education. There's got to be a commitment to actually access that health care if they're going to maintain any of it. If they've actually made the effort to go to a 'stop smoking' clinic the chances of them doing that are fairly workable. They've not come from a standpoint of having that imposed on them.
>
> (Collette, HP2)

Despite the positive presentation of such approaches in the media and health professional press (see, for example, Deville-Almond 1998, 2000; Browne 2000), the construction of drinking in pubs with friends as being representative of 'hedonistic escape' (see Chapter 4) by men means that discussing health in such a setting is almost antithetical. As Martin suggests:

> You read in the paper about setting up GP surgeries in pubs, a load of rubbish. Men are just gonna stand there and laugh at them with a pint. I can't see that sort of tact of working at all [. . .] Your pub's your greatest escape innit? You don't wanna be told that you're ill, you wanna few drinks with your mates and a good laugh.
>
> (Martin, CABS3)

A different opportunity was felt to be afforded by considering the health of men in the workplace. Seven of the men and two health professionals spontaneously identified work as a suitable place for health promotion with men, and three recounted positive experiences of encounters of such nature. The potential shape of suggested projects varied from the provision of health information, through well-man checks, to having established exercise programmes available, although there was recognition that employers would have to be seen to benefit, or at least not lose out financially, through such arrangements:

> The workplace would be quite a good idea for targeting people. Provide some incentive for the firms themselves to do that for the workers; exercise programmes and that. Sort of, you know, an hour off. But I suppose the bosses would have to have an incentive to hold that sort of thing, money is the only thing that talks in business.
>
> (Gary, GM3)

This tightening business culture was also seen to present other possible problems to such initiatives, with some men being concerned that health information collected or gained through such schemes may be used for punitive purposes:

> We've got the Occupational Health Service and of course that's getting a lot tougher. In the past you could be off for six or seven weeks and they wouldn't bother. Now if you're off for three weeks they're ringing you up, or sending somebody round to see you. A few years ago that happened to me at work. I got referred to a doctor there [occupational health] and he basically warned me, he really scared me in a way, he said 'Well if you don't get your bloody act together you'll be out of here'. As I say it's all pressure now.
>
> (Francis, CABS1)

The potential for occupational health to be seen as having a 'policing' role, and therefore viewed with suspicion as a provider of health services, and financial concerns about implementing such services, have been noted in some previous research looking at health promotion for men in the workplace (Summer et al. 2002). Given the continued (though possibly reducing) importance of work in the construction of (hegemonic) masculinity (Haywood and Mac an Ghaill 2003: 19*ff*), it is not surprising that the type of services discussed by the men were NHS-provided services that came independently to the workplace rather than being workplace provided. Nevertheless, as was found in other research (Dolan et al. 2005), health promotion in the workplace does seem to be received positively by men.

The recognition of GP surgeries as 'feminized' space, combined with a hegemonic male desire to maintain control, led several men to suggest that one-to-one sessions in their own homes, where they have time in a safe setting to discuss their health concerns, was a potential way forward for health promotion work with men:

> You know consultation where they call and see you. I would say you need to do what you're doing now, come and see me and to talk with me, listen to me, and then come up with an idea. That would be a good thing. Safe environment, comfortable environment, where there is no shocks, no hidden punches, nothing major at first, they just lead you into it calmly and win your confidence like a pat on the back approach, yeah.
>
> (Dan, CABS7)

Face to face?

For many, this linked with an idea that privacy and confidentiality were of key importance to men. In this respect, anonymous modes of communication, particularly telephone and Internet services, were also suggested as creating new opportunities for desirable models of health contact with men:

> *SR:* Where would men feel safe going with that [health] issue?
> *Martin:* I think the telephone would probably be one of the only ways men would do it. They feel a bit more secure over the telephone, they don't have to talk to someone about it, the telephone, the Internet even I guess [...] I think it's because it's an anonymous thing.
>
> (Martin, CABS3)

Such approaches were seen to help maintain a high degree of control and independence and also negate what can be the potentially problematic area of engaging in physical encounters. As such, these models are increasingly being recognized by health professionals as providing one way forward in health promotion work with men (Robertson and Williams 1997; Davidson 2001; Fletcher 2001).

However, it is obviously not always possible to maintain distance in medical encounters, particularly when the men felt that the breakdown of physiological processes demanded health professional intervention. Narratives regarding such direct encounters, perhaps not surprisingly, were most common in the interviews with the disabled men and those men with chronic illnesses, many of whom had developed ongoing relationships with health professionals (mainly GPs and specialist consultants). These narratives tended to follow a pattern, being characterized by the men as consisting of initial (power) struggles that evolved into a relationship based on trust and mutual respect:

> It's all wrong because they're employing staff not capable of communicating, like [consultant] when he told me I had to have me leg off. I'm always a joker, so I had someone draw me a picture of Long John Silver, 'I'm getting leg-less on Thursday.' He come round and flipped, 'I'm not doing your operation, you've got the wrong attitude.' [laugh]. So I said, 'if you talk into that Dictaphone anymore, and talk to the sister, I'll shove that Dictaphone right up your arse.' I says, 'Speak to me, I'm the patient.' The next time he comes round, he has his Dictaphone, put it away, and I said, 'That's right talk to me, don't talk to that Dictaphone.' Ever since that we've got on really well.
>
> (Vernon, DM4)

Such power struggles, and the role that current gender structures played in them, were also recognized by the health professionals as being significant in the way lay–professional interactions proceeded:

> SR: Do you think, generally speaking, men are more anxious than women about going to the GP?
>
> Collette: Yeah. I don't really know why but I think it's more of an irritation for them. Women, as women, perhaps tend to be more easily put in a situation of hierarchical order. They're quite happy to sit and wait at the GPs and don't really question too much whereas a man would sort of look for a more egalitarian situation and therefore would challenge any action they're not comfortable with [laughs].
>
> (Collette, HP2)

For the men, these processes were linked both to initial difficulties in relinquishing (some) control, which usually required being convinced of the individual health professional's knowledge and capabilities, and overcoming the (homosexual) connotations associated with physical touch. As Bob makes clear:

> Now I'm used to the doctor cause I've been with my MS. But when it first happened, it was like blood out of a stone with me, 'Why do you want to know these things, is there something wrong with me, tell me if there's something wrong with me!' And there's these probing questions, this investigative line that they were taking with me, and I felt very defensive. I thought, whoa, whoa, whoa, why are you asking me all this stuff? I wanted to make sure they were qualified to ask me

these things. At one point I said, 'Show me your badge. I want to know that you're qualified to ask me these questions.' Putting my barrier up, even to the, you know, 'open your shirt'. I think men are naturally homophobic, 'Why?' 'I want to listen to your heart'. 'Oh, all right.' And even the doctor when he said, 'Well, drop your trousers.' OK, [cough] let's be men about this, you know. But I think yeah, men are very naturally homophobic, they just don't like anything too far out of the ordinary.

(Bob, CABS6)

Whilst some previous work (Howard 1996) suggests that such homophobia leads men to prefer female health professionals, accounts here, and in other recent research (Lomas 2003), suggest that the situation is more complex than this. In line with previous research (Kerssens et al. 1997), female (health professional) skills in listening were often stated as being important by the men when problems were ones that required discussion rather than straightforward diagnosis and treatment:

I prefer to see a lady doctor. At my practice there's one lady doctor and three guy doctors, and I normally say 'Can I book an appointment to see [lady doctor]', because she's really nice, she's lovely, and if I'm telling people things, I prefer to speak to her than I would the other fellas. I would go and see her.

(David, GM1)

Yet, the way that emotion is often understood as being action-orientated for men (outlined in Chapter 4) means that the need for practical input and support can itself be what creates trust and, over time, helps develop relationships with specific health professionals:

My GP is fantastic. This is somebody from before my accident, a family doctor, only a young gentleman and he is just awesome, absolutely awesome. If I've got any problems I don't have to worry. He's even been on courses to do with spinal injuries and things and he's just fantastic, I can't ask for a better GP. You get to trust certain doctors and I know that if I have any problems, or I need more information, or advice or whatever, then he's more than happy, and if he doesn't know it himself he'll look it up or will find out for me.

(Peter, DM1)

This in itself creates a situation where the space for confiding becomes available and this is no longer dependent on the gender of the health professional *once a relationship, initially built on practical need, is established*:

SR: If you were to try and define the things that made it a good rela-
          tionship what would they be?

Frank: It's the things you have to tell your GP, you can never tell anybody
          else. Yeah, you've told him really bad things so, I think it makes you
          more relaxed towards them. I went to the GP with a lump in me
          chest, and I was terrified, and he was really good, yeah he was. I think
          that's why I stayed with his practice for so long because he was really
          good [. . .] The only time I saw another doctor was when he was ill or
          on holiday or something. I never saw another doctor out of my
          choice, it was always because of something else.

                                                                    (Frank, DM6)

Women were felt to have an advantage here as their relationships with
GPs were seen to already be well developed through the regular contact they
had for cervical screening, contraception, and pregnancy and so forth.

In the same way, the screening for sexually transmitted diseases that was
a regular aspect of the gay men's lives also meant that relationships had
developed with health professionals over time. However, these relationships
had also been characterized by struggles and all the gay men interviewed had
experienced what they felt were homophobic attitudes from health service
staff at some point:

> Before I moved, I told my doctor that I was gay. Every time I saw him,
> for a bad back, breathing problem or whatever, he seemed to treat me
> totally different after that, and my perception of that is that he was
> homophobic and didn't like me because I was gay. I never tackled
> him about it, but as far as I am concerned, he was homophobic to
> me, even though he didn't even say it, I had those vibes off him.
>
>   (David, GM1)

As identified in previous research (Cant 1999), such experiences required
that special consideration be given when thinking about choosing and confiding in primary health care professionals about one's sexual identity as a gay
man. For some gay men these encounters had prompted a change of GP and
knowledge residing in the gay community about 'gay friendly' GPs was drawn
on at these times to facilitate this process. For others, the perceived significance of being seen was more important than the negative aspects of the
encounter, although as Gary shows, it affects the nature of the contact:

> I don't like him [doctor] at all. I think he's homophobic and because
> you're HIV positive you're dirt, or it seems to come over that way
> when he talked. Before I got diagnosed with HIV I used to go for a six-
> monthly check-up. And I really didn't like going if he was there, it

put me off going. *But I still went because I thought it was important* but I didn't like going because of him being there. Like I say he's very homophobic. I actually told him at first that I was heterosexual because I knew his views and was a bit worried about that.

(Gary, GM3, emphasis added)

Summary

Men's engagement with health services is clearly a complex process that is not sufficiently explained through reductionist notions of male stoicism and refusal to be seen as weak. The strong dichotomy maintained by the men between 'health' and 'illness' formed a key base for maintaining a distance from health information or services that were perceived as a potential threat to autonomy and control by their involvement in aspects of men's daily lives. Yet this dichotomy also allowed men to be seen, by themselves and health professionals, as 'serious' users of health services and therefore maintained legitimate access at times when physiological processes were seen to have broken down or appeared vulnerable.

A hegemonic masculine representation of health (not illness) as being a female domain or field further impacts on how health promotion or 'well-men' services are perceived by both men and health professionals. Hegemonic masculine values are both built into health service structures and serve to replicate these gendered structures. Thus, the identification of health as a female domain leads to the development of GP services that become seen as feminized spaces, giving the (further) impression that health is a feminized domain. In this way, as part of acquired sets of generative dispositions, hegemonic masculine values are both structured and structuring or structuring structures; they are both built into health service structures and serve in turn to replicate the gendered nature of the health service (Bourdieu 1990: 52*ff*; Williams 1995). Masculine representations have material effects, in this situation GP surgeries that become promulgated with female-orientated health promotion literature and services (see also Banks 2001).

Health promotion critiques based on the rise of surveillance medicine often fail to appreciate the subtle complexities of this relationship between gendered lay understanding(s) of health and the utilization of health information and screening services. The current hegemonic, patriarchal context that has seen the rise of surveillance medicine has specifically led to women becoming the focus of the instruments of disciplinary power (though women are far from passive victims of this process – see Howson 1998), creating the potential for men to be obfuscated by health promotion and screening services. This obfuscation enables men to avoid health professional interference in everyday life but creates clear dilemmas when physiological processes are seen as 'at risk' or vulnerable. At such times, varied means of legitimating access to health promotion, screening services were mobilized by the men. Specifically adopting or relying on a non-hegemonic masculine identity was one such strategy. This could be done through identifying as gay, through presenting a reformed disabled masculine identity, or even through a new hegemonic masculine identification as being disaffected with old hegemonic values.

Yet, such overt rejection of hegemonic masculine norms also carries the threat of being marginalized or subordinated from the material privileges associated with being at the top of the gender hierarchy. Alternative strategies were therefore also apparent. These included increasing the importance of privacy, confidentiality and anonymity in service provision (lessening the likelihood of anyone noticing the non-adherence to hegemonic values); relying on the 'nagging' of (female) partners, family or friends (thus replicating the idea that women are responsible for health and sustaining a hegemonic identity oneself); and identifying 'risk' to be at a level that not seeking help would be seen as irrational (replicating the hegemonic construction of masculinity as being inherently rational).

In these respects, despite the strong gendering of health and health promotion services as being a female domain, men showed themselves as markedly adept at creating a range of strategies, some outright resistance, others a reliance on hegemonic values, to facilitate access to health information, screening, and other health promoting services, at times when they felt this to be necessary. Whilst health professionals clearly recognized the difficulties for men that the feminization of health creates, future health promotion work would benefit from a more explicit understanding of, and working with, the strategies that men already use to facilitate access.

Key points

- Accepting individual responsibility for health can be a way for men to maintain autonomy, independence and control and so limit health professional 'interference'.
- Health professionals often perceived health education/promotion and 'lifestyle' advice approaches in primary care to be ineffective for men.
- Men saw the primary function of health services as treating those who were unwell; health promotion was seen as a secondary role for the NHS if resources permitted.
- Health 'screening' seemed to sit uneasily between the 'health/ ill-health' distinction that the men held.
- Being 'hidden' as health service users removed men from the 'medical gaze' but caused concern that harmful changes to physiological processes may be missed.

- Men have to legitimize engagement with health services and they can and do find various ways to do this.
- Relationships of trust can and do develop over time when health professionals help men meet situations of practical (instrumental) need.

Key points for practitioners

- Practitioners should not assume that men have an irresponsible attitude toward their health. Men are often clear that lifestyle choices are their responsibility and this can link closely with a need to be or feel in control.
- Men's distinction between who has responsibility for health and ill health suggests that health promoting activities may be best delivered outside of traditional health services structures and organizations though attention needs to be paid to the gendered nature of alternate venues.
- Screening for early detection of physiological changes disrupts this health/ill-health dichotomy and can create an opportunity for health promotion work with men.
- Men are often keen to have information about early signs and symptoms that may indicate underlying concerns but are not always keen on 'lifestyle advice' which can be seen as being told what to do.
- Practitioners could learn more about what legitimates engagement with health services or health promoting activities for men and use this to facilitate interaction.

Notes

1. This can still be the case when the individual health professional involved is female as power is still being exerted to serve patriarchal purposes (Davies 1995).
2. This changed for a short period later with the advent of National Service where such hierarchical observation and examination played a pivotal role in establishing and maintaining power relations.

6   Some conclusions

Introduction

Unlike the field of men and illness where there is a significant and growing body of qualitative research exploring men's experiences, there has been little previous work on men and health, and the relationship(s) between masculinity/masculinities and health, that are grounded in men's own accounts. In this book I have drawn on primary research data – lay men's and health professionals' own narrative accounts – and I have explored this with the help of previous empirical and theoretical work in order to learn more about how relationships between 'masculinities' and 'health practices' are shaped within, and by, particular social contexts. This movement between primary source accounts, theory, and existing empirical data is not always easy to achieve. This concluding chapter therefore reiterates the main points of significance and the links between these, while also suggesting what some of the practical implications of these might be, and highlighting potential areas for future research. In doing so it completes the circle by reintegrating the emerging points of theoretical and empirical significance back into the men's health research, policy and practice context.

Masculinity and conceptualizing men's health

Modern concerns about the health of men are often premised on men's reduced longevity (compared to women) and high rates of some male morbidity, particularly prostate and testicular cancers, liver disease and suicide. These are not seen as isolated epidemiological artefacts but are usually linked directly to aspects of men's 'behaviour', for instance alcohol and cigarette consumption, violence and inability to disclose emotionally, reluctance to attend health services and a greater propensity to take a variety of 'risks'. All of these are said to account for sex differences in health outcomes between men and women. 'Being a man', the social practices associated with 'masculinity', are therefore implicated in the creation of men's (usually poorer) health outcomes. These concerns, including the links made to masculinity, have been recognized explicitly at government level in the UK since the early 1990s and service providers tasked with doing more to address men's health needs. This government rhetoric, and increased media attention, have led to a greater number of services for men, including a rise in innovative health promotion projects, but there is still concern that these services are only having minimal impact on men's health outcomes and that lack of a firmer national governmental steer means that such services are often ad hoc, uncoordinated and financially vulnerable compared to other competing health priorities.

Part of the difficulty here is that simplistic assumptions are made about 'masculinity' and its relations to health practices and outcomes. Men are often homogenized within the rhetoric that surrounds the men's health field. They are frequently portrayed either as products of their genetic or hormonal processes, or as vessels socialized with a shared set of traits characteristic of appropriate male 'behaviours'. Either way, there is seen to be an essential, individual core that represents (and constrains) 'how *all* men are' (or at least how they are meant to be) and it is this that is said to promote risk taking and reduce help seeking amongst men. Yet, recent qualitative research has begun to question such simplistic assumptions, suggesting instead that men are far more diverse than this in their range of 'masculinity' and health-related practices, and demonstrating how such practices are contingent on sets of social circumstances (for example, O'Brien et al. 2005; McVittie and Willock 2006). This research reiterates the importance of understanding 'masculinity' as something created and realized through and within sets of relationships, and that these gendered relations are hierarchically ordered, becoming embedded in, and replicated through, social structures. In this sense, there are a range of 'masculinities', which can be seen as configurations of practice – most notably Connell's (1987, 1995) notions of hegemonic, subordinated, marginalized and complicit configurations – that men move within and between. To date, though, little work has been completed to look at how men's movement within and between these hierarchical configurations of practice relates to health practices and how varied social contexts mediate these relations.

The accounts provided here support previous research that highlights how men rarely reflect on 'health' as an abstract concept but rather understand and experience it as part of everyday life, and as part of a pragmatic embodiment (Watson 2000). It appears that men *qua* men (men as men, because they are men) are expected to have a 'don't care' attitude to health yet, as good citizens, are also expected to take responsibility for their health; that is, to have a 'should care' approach. This 'don't care/should care' dichotomy coalesces with thinking in late modernity that health promotion practices consist of both 'control' and 'release' and that having a 'blowout' has become as important as exercising 'restraint' in the project of maintaining 'good health' (Crawford 1984). Particular discourses, and actions, of 'don't care' or 'should care', and of 'control' or 'release', were combined in the men's accounts and used as a means of demonstrating, or specifically resisting and not demonstrating, hegemonic masculine values. What emerges then is a framework, shown as Figure 2.1 on p. 61 in Chapter 2, for explaining how the relationship between 'masculinity' and 'health' is played out in everyday life.

The tension created through this 'don't care/should care' dichotomy was not felt equally by all men, or was certainly managed in different ways in different situations. Gay masculinities, through an alignment with feminine values of care, concern and because of the personal experiences with HIV/AIDS, permitted (even obliged) gay men to take a 'should care' approach to health and well-being, although in practice this was often restricted to sexual health and well-being. Likewise, disabled men could use their impairment as a legitimate reason for caring about their health and well-being although this ran the risk of being emasculating and care was often taken in such narratives to reinsert a commitment to alternate hegemonic masculine values through notions such as 'edgework' (Collinson 1996; Lyng 2005); living dangerously without going 'too far'. Given the centrality of identity to managing this 'don't care/should care' dichotomy, it is envisaged that the influence of other masculinities configurations associated with ethnicity, age, socio-economic position, and so forth, will provide fertile and necessary areas for future research.

The relationship between 'risk' and 'responsibility' also provides insights into the socially contingent nature of men's health practices. Unlike much of the health professional literature that postulates men as irresponsible risk takers, accounts here show that 'risk' was more often a measured activity for the men frequently undertaken to offset other, seemingly more significant, 'risks'. There was an almost tacit understanding that the risks attached to hedonistic behaviour were worthwhile, or at least necessary, in order to reduce the risk of being socially isolated for younger men but that such hedonistic risk taking did, or ought to, reduce for the men as they settled into 'responsible' longer term relationships and particularly following becoming a father. In recognizing that men face a 'should care' aspect to their health practices, and that the taking of risks is also balanced with the desire to exercise responsible self-control, health practitioners can start to see (and seize) opportunities for promoting change based in men's everyday experiences rather than just focusing on the physiological or on trying to alter behaviour outside its social context.

Bodies and relationships in men's health

A narrow physiological or biomedical focus can reinforce a mechanistic view of men's bodies that fails to realize how men can and do listen to, and learn from, their own bodily experiences and those of others. Accounts here have helped expand Watson's (2000) previous work on health and the male body by looking more closely at how physiological, experiential and pragmatic embodiment are related. Contra recent trends in some postmodernist writing (Fox 1993), the 'healthy' body was necessarily understood by the men as *both* representational *and* material and a complex relationship between physiological, experiential and pragmatic embodiment was posited. There was recognition that real physiological processes underpinned the ability to function in everyday life (pragmatic embodiment) and that experiential embodiment (both one's own and that of those close) was key to both improving or maintaining these physiological process, in recognising when such process may be breaking down, and thereby in optimizing pragmatic functioning. The representation of masculine identity through embodied forms based on action and strength becomes problematic if changes such as physical impairment or chronic illness make this difficult to sustain. Rather than assuming a mechanistic view, health practitioners would benefit from learning how best to elicit and explore men's lived experiences in order to see where opportunity for change has good fit with men's daily lives.

The nature of the relationship between physiological, experiential and pragmatic embodiment in acute and chronic illness has begun to be explored (although studies do not tend to refer to it in this way), but further research with men looking at this same relationship during minor illness would be of value in considering how men manage the interface between health and illness and the implications of this for 'staying well', or promoting health, in everyday life (as opposed to considering how men come to terms with more severe and/or chronic ill-health).

The importance of understanding lived experiences also requires recognizing how healthy (male) bodies are as much a product of healthy public places and spaces as they are of individual behaviour(s) or physiology. As hegemonic configurations of practice become embedded in social structures, particular places become marked out as gendered spaces from which 'others' – women, children and non-hegemonic men – become marginalized. Such marginalization can have an impact on access to the material resources required to maximize well-being. It is important therefore when working towards improving men's health that practitioners try to understand which places and spaces facilitate or inhibit 'healthy practices' and what can be done to utilize or influence these circumstances.

The way that health is embedded in daily life also has resonance when thinking about the role of social connections, relationships, in men's lives. The feelings involved in close, sexual relationships were seen to be generative of 'good health' when going well and this was often because of 'natural' changes – usually termed 'settling down' and involving less hedonistic socialising and an improved diet – that occurred as the relationship developed. It is no surprise then that breakdown of these intimate relations seemed to create instability, a significant loss of purpose and place in the world (*existential angst*), that specifically necessitated a (re)negotiation of male identity and could return the men, if only temporarily, to those more hedonistic social practices. Parents remained an important and significant source of practical and emotional support for the men. Yet, this separation of the 'practical' from the 'emotional' was itself challenged by the accounts here. It was often engagement in practical tasks, either as recipient or provider, that generated deeper emotional bonds for the men and in this sense emotion is integrated into action. This was not just the case in relations with parents but also applied to men's friendships where shared (usually sustained) instrumental action created the necessary conditions for communicative action, including emotional confiding. Emotions, feeling, therefore become an integral part of doing; practical action becomes constitutive and generative of emotional intimacy in relationships for men. Love, hate and other emotions are recognized and realized through actions, not merely felt or discussed. The more precise nature of this embodied emotionality would clearly benefit from further empirical explication. Discussion generated here in Chapter 4 could be fruitfully applied (and further refined) to future research focused on gender, social connectedness and health where others have begun to recognize that previous work has tended to operate with a 'feminine ruler' when considering the quantity and quality of social networks and relationships and how these impact on health (Arber and Davidson 2002).

For practitioners, recognizing emotion *as* action becomes crucial in understanding how trust is developed and therefore how space for communicative action ('emotional confiding') can be created in health work with men. This has particular implications for the delivery of mental health services. It seems likely that situating therapeutic mental health work in action-based rather than communication-based models, at least in the early stages, is more likely to engage men and develop the trust needed to facilitate verbal communication, and some projects have begun to work successfully with men in this way (Melluish and Bulmer 1999; Borg 2002).

Responsibility and accessing health services

The men also made a strong distinction between 'health' and 'ill-health' that has implications for their use of services. The prime function of health services, particularly the National Health Service, was seen to be in treating those who are 'unwell'. Maintaining or promoting good health were seen as being the responsibility of the individual, or possibly as a secondary role for the NHS once they had met their 'ill-health' role and if resources then permitted. Shifting the responsibility for staying well back to the individual allowed the men to maintain control, autonomy and to avoid what could be seen as medical interference in everyday life. It creates opportunities for men to demonstrate both a 'don't care' discourse, by rejecting health advice, and a 'should care' discourse, by claiming themselves as independently responsible for their health. Screening services seemed to disrupt this 'health/ill-health' distinction. There was an understanding that pathological changes could take place, unrecognized by the experiential body, which could be detected by health professionals performing 'checks' and this could lead to early intervention and better health outcomes. Yet, there was also a feeling that screening services, although acceptable for women, required a degree of relinquishing of autonomy, control, and a submission to the 'medical gaze', which the men found unfamiliar and therefore difficult. Being 'hidden' from health promotion services in this way allowed men to avoid medical interference in their everyday life but also caused concern about possible harmful changes to physiological processes that may be missed.

The 'health/ill-health' distinction also prompted suggestions about delivering health promoting activities for men outside of traditional health services structures and organizations that tended to be viewed as 'feminized' spaces. Pubs, clubs and bars were recognized as places where such 'outreach' had already commenced but the equating of these spaces with hedonistic release was seen to limit the effectiveness, and even appropriateness, of health work in such venues. Workplaces, on the other hand, were seen as spaces offering great potential for health work with men, although it was important that this be delivered independently rather than through occupational health services who might be used as 'policing agents' by employers. The increased anonymity offered by telephone helplines and Internet-based services was also thought to make these potentially attractive forums for health promotion with men. It is clear that not all innovative work in alternative settings was equally valued and it is important for health practitioners to consider how particular places and spaces are gendered and how this may affect the accessibility for men of services delivered through these venues.

In all settings, it was apparent that men needed to legitimate their engagement with health services thus managing the 'don't care/should care' dichotomy; 'health' could not be done just for its own sake. Forms of legitimating included: observing ill-health in close friends or relatives; having a family history of particular health problems; having a level of injury/symptom/impairment where it was justified that not seeking help would be irrational; and being encouraged to go by significant others (usually female spouse or family member). This is not necessarily an exhaustive list and other aspects of identity not considered here, such as age, ethnicity, social class and so forth, may create other forms of legitimating that could be uncovered in future research. Practitioners can learn to recognize and utilize these process of legitimation in their endeavours to engage in health promotion work with men.

Final thoughts

Clearly this work has limitations. The primary research on which it draws is relatively small scale, completed in a specific geographical region of the UK, and did not include men of different ethnic groups or social classes. In this sense I have only been able to begin the process of looking at how relationships between 'masculinities' and 'health practices' are shaped within a limited number of social contexts, many more are yet to be explored. Nevertheless, the conceptual discussion of the issues involved, stimulated through the links made with previous theoretical and empirical work, give it a broader social resonance in places that share similar cultural, political and economic backgrounds.

Throughout this book, the detailed accounts provided, in interviews lasting up to three hours, challenge the preconceived, homogenizing notion that men will not, or cannot, talk and share experiences and particularly health-related experiences. It suggests, as others have also found (Brown 2001; Oliffe and Mróz 2005; Emslie et al. 2006), that given the right approach and circumstances, some men at least are very able to articulate aspects of their health experiences. These accounts and their interpretation illustrate the complexity of relationships between men, masculinities and health-related practices and make it clear that simplistic explanations equating men with *a* masculinity and masculinity with negative health practices and outcomes, bare little relation to men's diverse lived experiences. Yet, at the same time, these experiences are not so diverse and fragmented that they merely represent idiosyncratic accounts. It is possible in conceptualizing masculinities as hierarchical configurations of practice that men move within and between to begin to see how particular patterns of health practices are facilitated or inhibited for men in specific social contexts.

Exploring the complexity of relationships between masculinities, and particularly the relationship between hegemonic and subordinated and/or marginalized masculinities, demonstrates how these are then played out (and played with) in their relationship to health and well-being. Clearly, neither 'masculinity' or 'health' are static concepts and they can both take on, or be given, different meanings at different times by men as potential health service users and by health professionals as health service providers. In this sense, it is not only 'masculinity' that is present as these varied 'configurations of practice' that men move within and between (Connell 1995: 71*ff*). The array of language used – 'fitness', 'well-being', 'feeling good', 'looking good', 'ill', 'sick', 'infirm' – I would suggest is also representative of the naming of configurations of varied health-related practices that may also be hierarchically ordered and certainly have specific social (moral) values.

The work has also begun to show that, despite being fluid and fragmented concepts, both 'masculinity' and 'health' are not entirely incomplete and without substance. They are malleable and adaptable, allowing men to move within and between different configurations but they are not confused or incoherent. The hierarchical embedding of different configurations into social structures and social practices creates hegemonic forms of 'masculinity' and 'health' that gives representational and material preference to these forms. This representational and material privileging creates opportunities for those able and willing to engage in or be complicit with these hegemonic configurations. Likewise, it subordinates and marginalizes others, restricting opportunities (yet also offering sites of resistance), to those who are unwilling or unable to engage in, or be complicit with, hegemonic configurations. It is only through explicitly recognizing the importance of gendered identity, in individual action *and* in social structures, that one can begin to recognize how, when, where and why particular configurations of health practices emerge for men. It is essential that future research and health practitioners learn to problematize 'masculinity' and 'health' in this way if health work with men is to progress in a positive and sustainable direction for the benefit of all in society.

References

Acheson, D. (1998) *Inequalities in Health*. London: HMSO.

Adams, L., Amos, M. and Munro, J. (eds) (2002) *Promoting Health: Politics and Practice*. London: Sage.

Annandale, E. and Hunt, K. (1990) Masculinity, femininity and sex: an exploration of their relative contribution to explaining gender differences in health, *Sociology of Health and Illness*, 12(1): 24–45.

Annandale, E. and Hunt, K. (2000) Gender inequalities in health: research at the crossroads, in E. Annandale, K. Hunt (eds) *Gender Inequalities in Health*. Buckingham: Open University Press.

Arber, S. (1991) Class, paid employment and family roles: making sense of structural disadvantage, gender and health status, *Social Science and Medicine*, 32: 425–36.

Arber, S. (1997) Comparing inequalities in women's and men's health: Britain in the 1990s, *Social Science and Medicine*, 44(6): 773–87.

Arber, S. and Cooper, H. (2000) Gender and inequalities in health across the lifecourse, in E. Annandale, K. Hunt (eds) *Gender Inequalities in Health*. Buckingham: Open University Press.

Arber, S. and Davidson, K. (2002) *Older Men: their Social Worlds and Healthy Lifestyles*. Guildford: Centre for Research on Ageing and Gender (CRAG), University of Surrey.

Armstrong, D. (1983) *Political Anatomy of the Body*. Cambridge: Cambridge University Press.

Armstrong, D. (1995) The rise of surveillance medicine, *Sociology of Health and Illness*, 17(3): 393–404.

Backett, K. and Davison, C. (1995) Lifecourse and lifestyle: the social and cultural location of health behaviours, *Social Science and Medicine*, 40(5): 629–38.

Baggot, R. (2000) *Public Health: Policy and Politics*. Basingstoke: Macmillan Press.

Banks, I. (2001) No mans land: men, illness and the NHS, *British Medical Journal*, 323: 1058–60.

Banks, I. (2004) New models for providing men with health care, *Journal of Men's Health and Gender*, 1(2/3): 155–8.

Beattie, A. (1991) Knowledge and control in health promotion: a test case for social policy and social theory, in J. Gabe, M. Calnan and M. Bury (eds) *The Sociology of the Health Service*. London: Routledge.

Bem, S. (1974) The measurement of psychological androgyny, *Journal of Consulting and Clinical Psychology*, 42(2): 155–62.

Bem, S. (1981) *Bem Sex-role Inventory Professional Manual*. Palo Alto: Consulting Psychologists Press.

Bennett, M. (1995) Why don't men come to counselling? Some speculative theories, *Counselling*, 6: 44–8.

Blaxter, M. (1990) *Health and Lifestyles*. London: Routledge.

Blaxter, M. (1997) Whose fault is it? People's own conceptions of the reasons for health inequalities, *Social Science and Medicine*, 44(6): 747–56.

Blaxter, M. and Paterson, E. (1982) *Mothers and Daughters: A Three-Generational Study of Health Attitudes and Behaviour*. London: Heinemann.

Bloor, M. (1995) *The Sociology of HIV Transmission*. London: Sage.

Bloor, M. and McIntosh, J. (1990) Surveillance and concealment: a comparison of techniques of client resistance in therapeutic communities and health visiting, in S. Cunningham-Burley and N. McKeganey (eds) *Readings in Medical Sociology*. London: Routledge.

Borg, M.B. (2002) The Avalon Gardens Men's Association: a community health psychology study, *Journal of Health Psychology*, 7(3): 345–57.

Boroughs, M. and Thompson, J.K. (2002) Body depilation in males: a new body image concern? *International Journal of Men's Health*, 1(3): 247–57.

Bourdieu, P. (1977) *Outline of a Theory of Practice*. Cambridge: Cambridge University Press.

Bourdieu, P. (1979) *Distinction: A Social Critique of the Judgement of Taste*. London: Routledge.

Bourdieu, P. (1990) *The Logic of Practice*. Cambridge: Polity Press.

Brannen, J., Dodd, K., Oakley, A. and Storey, P. (1994) *Young People, Health and Family Life*. Milton Keynes: Open University Press.

Brown, I. and Lunt, F. (1992) Evaluating a 'well man' clinic, *Health Visitor*, 65(1): 12–15.

Brown, S. (2001) What makes men talk about health? *Journal of Gender Studies*, 10(2): 187–95.

Browne, A. (2000) Men raise a glass to good health. *Observer*, 27 February.

Brownhill, S., Wilhelm, K., Barclay, L. and Schmied, V. (2005) 'Big build': hidden depression in men, *Australian and New Zealand Journal of Psychiatry*, 39: 921–31.

Buchbinder, D. (1998) A well-shaped man, in A. Petersen and C. Waddell (eds) *Health Matters: Sociology of Illness, Prevention and Care*. Buckingham: Open University Press.

Butler, J. (1993) *Bodies that Matter: On the Discursive Limits of 'Sex'*. London: Routledge.

Calnan, M. (1987) *Health and Illness: The Lay Perspective*. London: Tavistock.

Cameron, E. and Bernardes, J. (1998) Gender and disadvantage in health: men's health for a change, *Sociology of Health and Illness*, 20(5): 673–93.

Canaan, J.E. (1996) 'One thing leads to another': drinking, fighting and working class masculinities, in M. Mac an Ghaill (ed.) *Understanding Masculinities*. Buckingham: Open University Press.

Cancer Research UK (2006) UK prostate cancer incidence statistics. http://info. cancerresearchuk.org:8000/cancerstats/types/prostate/incidence/ (accessed 15 Dec. 2006).

Cant, B. (1999) *Primary Care and Gay and Bisexual Men*. Bromley: Bromley Health Authority.

Cantor, C.H. and Slater, P.J. (1995) Marital breakdown, parenthood and suicide, *Journal of Family Studies*, 1: 91–102.

Capraro, R.L. (2000) Why college men drink: alcohol, adventure and the paradox of masculinity, *Journal of American College Health*, 48: 307–15.

Carpenter, M. (2000) Reinforcing the pillars: rethinking gender, social divisions and health, in E. Annandale, K. Hunt (eds) *Gender Inequalities in Health*. Buckingham: Open University Press.

Carrigan, T., Connell, R.W. and Lee, J. (1985) Hard and heavy: toward a new sociology of masculinity, *Theory and Society*, 14: 551–603.

Carter, S. (1993) Risk masculinity and modernity: understandings of gender and danger in the modern period. Unpublished PhD thesis, Lancaster University.

Cascarino, T. (2003) The last taboo, *The Times*, Game-On sports section, 28 April

Castells, M. (1983) *The City and the Grass Roots*. London: Edward Arnold.

Caulfield, H. and Platzer, H. (1998) Next of kin, *Nursing Standard*, 13(7): 47–9.

Chalmers, K. (1991) Working with men: an analysis of health visiting practice in families with young children, *International Journal of Nursing Studies*, 29(1): 3–16.

Chapple, A. and Ziebland, S. (2002) Prostate cancer: embodied experience and perceptions of masculinity, *Sociology of Health and Illness*, 24(6): 820–41.

Charles, N. and Kerr, M. (1988) *Women, Food and Families*. Manchester: Manchester University Press.

Charmaz, K. (1995) Identity dilemmas of chronically ill men, in D. Sabo and D. F. Gordon (eds) *Men's Health and Illness: Gender, Power and the Body*. London: Sage.

Clare, A. (2001) *On Men: Masculinity in Crisis*. London: Arrow Books.

Clarke, S. and Popay, J. (1998) 'I'm just a bloke who has kids': men and women on parenthood, in J. Popay, J. Hearn and J. Edwards (eds) *Men, Gender Divisions and Welfare*. London: Routledge.

Clatterbaugh, K. (1990) *Contemporary Perspectives on Masculinity: Men, Women and Politics in Modern Society*. Oxford: Westview Press.

Clatterbaugh, K. (1998) What is problematic about masculinities? *Men and Masculinities*, 1(1): 24–45.

Cohen, T.F. (1992) Men's families, men's friends: a structural analysis of constraints on men's social ties, in P. Nardi (ed.) *Men's Friendships*. London: Sage.

Coleman, W. (1990) Doing masculinity/doing theory, in J. Hearn and D.H.J. Morgan (eds) *Men, Masculinities and Social Theory*. London: Unwin Hyman.

Collison, M. (1996) In search of the high life: drugs, crime, masculinities and consumption, *British Journal of Criminology*, 36(3): 428–44.

Connell, R.W. (1987) *Gender and Power: Society, the Person and Sexual Politics* Cambridge: Polity Press.

Connell, R.W. (1992) A very straight gay: masculinity, homosexual experience and the dynamics of gender, *American Sociological Review*, 57: 735–51.

Connell, R.W. (1995) *Masculinities*. Cambridge: Polity Press.

Connell, R.W. (1998) Masculinities and globalization, *Men and Masculinities*, 1(1): 3–23.

Connell, R.W. (2000) *The Men and the Boys*. Cambridge: Polity Press.

Connell, R.W., Davis, M.D. and Dowsett, G.W. (1993) A bastard of a life: homosexual desire and practice among men in working-class milieux, *Australia and New Zealand Journal of Sociology*, 29: 112–35.

Cornwall, A. and Lindisfarne, N. (eds) (1994) *Dislocating Masculinity: Comparative Ethnographies* London: Routledge.

Cornwell, J. (1984) *Hard-Earned Lives: Accounts of Health and Illness from East London*. London: Tavistock.

Courtenay, W.H. (2000a) Behavioural factors associated with disease, injury and death among men: evidence and implications for prevention, *Journal of Men's Studies*, 9(1): 81–142.

Courtenay, W.H. (2000b) Constructions of masculinity and their influence on men's well-being: a theory of gender and health, *Social Science and Medicine*, 50(10): 1385–401.

Cox, B.D., Huppert, F.A. and Whichelow, M.J. (1997) (eds) *The Health and Lifestyle Survey: Seven Years On*. Dartmouth: Aldershot.

Cramer, D.W. and Roach, A.J. (1988) Coming out to mom and dad: a study of gay males and their relationships with their parents, *Journal of Homosexuality*, 15(3/4): 79–91.

Crawford, R. (1980) Healthism and the medicalization of everyday life, *International Journal of Health Services*, 10(3): 365–88.

Crawford, R. (1984) A cultural account of health: control, release and the social body, in J.B. McKinlay (ed.) *Issues in the Political Economy of Health*. London: Tavistock.

Crawford, R. (2000) The ritual of health promotion, in S.J. Williams, J. Gabe and M. Calnan (eds) *Health, Medicine and Society: Key Theories, Future Agendas*. London: Routledge.

Crawford, R. (2006) Health as a meaningful social practice, *Health*, 10(4): 401–20.

Crossley, M.L. (2002) The perils of health promotion and the 'barebacking' backlash, *Health*, 6(1): 47–68.

Crossley, N. (1998) Emotion and communicative action: Habermas, linguistic philosophy and existentialism, in G. Bendelow and S.J. Williams (eds) *Emotions in Social Life: Critical Themes and Contemporary Issues*. London: Routledge.

Currer, C. (1986) Concepts of mental well- and ill-being: the case of Pathan mothers in Britain, in C. Currer, M. Stacey (eds) *Concepts of Health, Illness and Disease: A Comparative Perspective*. Leamington Spa: Berg.

Curry, T.J. (2000) Booze and bar fights: a journey to the dark side of college athletics, in J. McKay, M. Messner and D. Sabo (eds) *Masculinities, Gender Relations and Sport*. London: Sage.

Davidson, N. (2001) Guidelines for practice, in N. Davidson and T. Lloyd (eds) *Promoting Men's Health: A Guide for Practitioners*. London: Baillière Tindall.

Davidson, N. and Lloyd, T. (eds) (2001) *Promoting Men's Health: A Guide for Practitioners*. London: Baillière Tindall.

Davies, C. (1995) *Gender and the Professional Predicament in Nursing*. Buckingham, Open University Press.

Davison, C., Frankel, S. and Davey-Smith, G. (1992) The limits of lifestyle: reassessing fatalism in the popular culture of illness prevention, *Social Science and Medicine*, 34(6): 675–85.

Denton, M. and Walters, V. (1999) Gender differences in structural and behavioural determinants of health: an analysis of the social production of health, *Social Science and Medicine*, 48: 122–35.

Department of Health (1989) *General Practice in the National Health Service: The 1990 Contract*. London: HMSO.

Department of Health (1992) *The Health of the Nation*. London: HMSO.

Department of Health (1993) *On the State of Public Health 1992. The Annual Report of the Chief Medical Officer*. London: HMSO.

Department of Health (1999) *Saving Lives: Our Healthier Nation*. London: HMSO.

Department of Health (2000) *Health Minister to announce new plans to improve men's health: Yvette Cooper sets out action to tackle gender inequalities*. Press release, 29 March.

Department of Health (2003) *Tackling Health Inequalities: A Programme for Action*. London: HMSO.

Department of Health (2004) *Winterton urges men to use their pharmacies*. Press release, 2 April.

Deville-Almond, J. (1998) Power points, *Nursing Times*, 94(36): 32–4.

Deville-Almond, J. (2000) Man troubles, *Nursing Times*, 96(11): 28–9.

Dolan, A., Staples, V., Summer, S. and Hundt, G.L. (2005) 'You ain't going to say I've got a problem down there': workplace-based prostate health promotion with men, *Health Education Research*, 20(6): 730–8.

Donovan, J.L. (1986) *We Don't Buy Sickness, it Just Comes: Health, Illness and Health Care in the Lives of People in London*. Aldershot: Gower.

Doyal, L. (2000) Gender equity in health: debates and dilemmas, *Social Science and Medicine*, 51(6): 931–9.

Doyal, L. (2001) Sex, gender and health: the need for a new approach, *British Medical Journal*, 323: 1061–3.

Duncombe, J. and Marsden, D. (1993) Love and intimacy: the gender division of emotion and emotion work, *Sociology*, 27(2): 221–41.

Duncombe, J. and Marsden, D. (1998) 'Stepford wives' and 'hollow men'? Doing emotion work, doing gender and 'authenticity' in intimate heterosexual relationships, in G. Bendelow and S.J. Williams (eds) *Emotions in Social Life: Critical Themes and Contemporary Issues*. London: Routledge.

Dunnell, K., Fitzpatrick, J. and Bunting, J. (1999) Making use of official statistics in research on gender and health status: recent British data, *Social Science and Medicine*, 48(1): 117–27.

Emslie, C., Hunt, K. and Macintyre, S. (1999) Problematizing gender, work and health: the relationship between gender, occupational grade, working conditions and minor morbidity in full-time bank employees, *Social Science and Medicine*, 48(1): 33–48.

Emslie, C., Ridge, D., Ziebland, S. and Hunt, K. (2006) Men's accounts of depression: reconstructing or resisting hegemonic masculinity? *Social Science and Medicine*, 62(9): 2246–57.

Essex, C. (1996) Men's health: don't blame the victims, *British Medical Journal*, 312: 1040.

Fareed, A. (1994) Equal rights for men, *Nursing Times*, 90(5): 26–9.

Farrant, W. (1991) Addressing the contradictions: health promotion and community health action in the United Kingdom, *International Journal of Health Services*, 21(3): 423–39.

Fee, D. (2000) 'One of the guys': instrumentality and intimacy in gay men's friendships with straight men, in P. Nardi (ed.) *Gay Masculinities*. London: Sage.

Fletcher, R. (2001) The development of men's health in Australia, in N. Davidson and T. Lloyd (eds) (2001) *Promoting Men's Health: A Guide for Practitioners*. London: Baillière Tindall.

Flowers, P., Smith, J.A., Sheeran, P. and Beail, N. (1998) 'Coming out' and sexual debut: understanding the social context of HIV risk-related behaviour, *Journal of Community and Applied Social Psychology*, 8(6): 409–21.

Forrest, D. (1994) We're here, we're queer and we're not going shopping: changing gay male identities in contemporary Britain, in A. Cornwall and N. Lindisfarne (eds) *Dislocating Masculinity: Comparative Ethnographies*. London: Routledge.

Foucault, M. (1979) *Discipline and Punish: The Birth of the Prison*. Harmondsworth: Penguin.

Foucault, M. (1980) *Power/Knowledge*. Gordon, C. (ed.). Brighton: Harvester.

Fox, N. (1993) *Postmodernism, Sociology and Health*. Buckingham: Open University Press.

Fraser, D. (1984) *The Evolution of the British Welfare State: A History of Social Policy since the Industrial Revolution*. London: Macmillan Press.

Frosh, S., Phoenix, A. and Pattman, R. (2002) *Young Masculinities*. Basingstoke: Palgrave.

Fuhrer, R., Stansfeld, S.A., Chemali, J. and Shipley, M.J. (1999) Gender, social relations and mental health: prospective findings from an occupational cohort (Whitehall II study), *Social Science and Medicine*, 48: 77–87.

Galdas, P., Cheater, F. and Marshall, P. (2005) Men and help-seeking behaviour: literature review, *Journal of Advanced Nursing*, 49(6): 616–23.

Galvin, R. (2002) Disturbing notions of chronic illness and individual responsibility: towards a genealogy of morals, *Health*, 6(2): 107–37.

Gannon, K., Glover, L., O'Neill, M. and Emberton, M. (2004) Men and chronic illness: a qualitative study of LUTS, *Journal of Health Psychology*, 9(3): 411–20.

Gardner, J. and Oswald, A. (2002) *Is it Money or Marriage that Keeps People Alive?* Coventry: Department of Economics, University of Warwick.

Gerschick, T.J. and Miller, A.S. (1995) Coming to terms: masculinity and physical disability, in D. Sabo and D.F. Gordon (eds) *Men's Health and Illness: Gender, Power and the Body*. London: Sage.

Giddens, A. (1992) *The Transformation of Intimacy: Love Sexuality and Eroticism in Modern Societies*. Cambridge: Polity Press.

Ginsburg, N. (1992) *Divisions of Welfare: A Critical Introduction to Comparative Social Policy*. London: Sage.

Goffman, E. (1968) *Stigma: Some Notes on the Management of Spoiled Identity*. Harmondsworth: Penguin.

Goffman, E. (1969) *The Presentation of Self in Everyday Life*. Harmondsworth: Penguin.

Gordon, D.F. (1995) Testicular cancer and masculinity, in D. Sabo and D.F. Gordon (eds) *Men's Health and Illness: Gender, Power and the Body*. London: Sage.

Gough, B. (2006) Try to be healthy but don't forgo your masculinity: deconstructing men's health discourse in the media, *Social Science and Medicine*, 63(9): 2476–88.

Gough, B. and Edwards, G. (1998) The beer talking: four lads, a carry out and the reproduction of masculinities, *The Sociological Review*, 46(3): 409–35.

Graham, H. (1987) Women's smoking and family health, *Social Science and Medicine*, 25(1): 47–56.

Gray, R.E. (2003) *Prostate Tales: Men's Experiences with Prostate Cancer*. Harriman TN: Men's Studies Press.

Griffiths, S. (1996) Men's health: unhealthy lifestyles and an unwillingness to seek medical help, *British Medical Journal*, 312: 69–70.

Griffiths, S. (1999) Men as risk takers, in R.S. Kirby, M.G. Kirby and R.N. Farah (eds) *Men's Health*. Oxford: Isis Medical Media.

Griffiths, S. (2001) Inequalities in men's health, in N. Davidson and T. Lloyd (eds) *Promoting Men's Health: A Guide for Practitioners*. London: Baillière Tindall.

Grogan, S. and Richards, H. (2002) Body image; focus groups with boys and men, *Men and Masculinities*, 4(3): 219–32.

Gutterman, D.S. (1994) Postmodernism and the interrogation of masculinity, in H. Brod and M. Kaufman (eds) *Theorizing Masculinities*. London: Sage.

Hallert, C., Sandlund, O. and Broqvist, M. (2003) Perceptions of health-related quality of life of men and women living with ceoliac disease, *Scandinavian Journal of Caring Sciences*, 17: 301–7.

Hammond, P. (1994) Men's bits, *Nursing Times*, 90(16): 64.

Hammond, P. (2000) Blinkered views that hurt men, *Daily Express*, 25 January.

Harding, J. (1997) Bodies at risk: sex, surveillance and hormone replacement therapy, in A. Peterson and R. Bunton (eds) *Foucault, Health and Medicine*. London: Routledge.

Harré, R. (1991) *Physical Being: A Theory for a Corporeal Psychology*. Oxford: Basil Blackwell.

Hart, G., Fitzpatrick, R., McLean, J., Dawson, J. and Boulton, M. (1990) Gay men, social support and HIV disease: a study of social integration in the gay community, *AIDS Care*, 2: 163–70.

Hart, G. and Flowers, P. (2001) Gay and bisexual men's general health, in N. Davidson and T. Lloyd (eds) *Promoting Men's Health: A Guide for Practitioners*. London: Baillière Tindall.

Haywood, C. and Mac An Ghaill, M. (2003) *Men and Masculinities: Theory, Research and Social Practice*. Buckingham: Open University Press.

Hearn, J. (1993) Emotive subjects: organisational men, organisational masculinities and the (de)construction of emotions, in S. Fineman (ed.) *Emotion in Organisations*. London: Sage.

Hearn, J. and Morgan, D.H.J. (eds) (1990) *Men, Masculinities and Social Theory*. London: Unwin Hyman.

Helgeson, V.S. (1995) Masculinity, men's roles, and coronary heart disease, in D. Sabo and D.F. Gordon (eds) *Men's Health and Illness: Gender, Power and the Body*. London: Sage.

Henwood, K., Gill, R. and McLean, C. (2002) The changing man, *Psychologist*, 15(4): 182–6.

Herzlich, C. (1973) *Health and Illness*. London: Academic Press.

Hey, V. (1986) *Patriarchy and Pub Culture*. London: Tavistock Publications.

Higgs, P. (1998) Risk, governmentality and the reconceptualisation of citizenship, in G. Scramble and P. Higgs (eds) *Modernity, Medicine and Health*. London: Routledge.

Hobbs, A. (1995) Shattering the myths of masculinity, *Healthlines*, July/August, pp. 14–16.

Holroyd, G. (2002) Silent cries: reflections on men's health promotion, in L. Jones, M. Sidell and J. Douglas (eds) *The Challenge of Promoting Health: Exploration and Action* (2nd edn). Buckingham: Open University Press.

Home Office (2005) *Criminal Statistics England and Wales 2004*. London: Home Office.

Home Office (2006) *Crime in England and Wales 2005–6*. London: Home Office Statistical Bulletin.

Howard, W. (1996) *Men's Attitudes to Health Checks and Awareness of Male-specific Cancers*. London: Health Education Authority.

Howlett, B.C., Ahmad, W.I. and Murray, R. (1992) An exploration of White, Asian and Afro-Caribbean peoples' concepts of health and illness causation, *New Community*, 18(2): 281–92.

Howson, A. (1998) Embodied obligation: the female body and health surveillance, in S. Nettleton and J. Watson (eds) *The Body in Everyday Life*. London: Routledge.

Hughner, R.S. and Kleine, S.S. (2004) Views of health in the lay sector: a compilation and review of how individuals think about health, *Health*, 8(4): 395–422.

Hunt, K., Davison, C., Emslie, C. and Ford, G. (2000a) Are perceptions of family history of heart disease related to health-related attitudes and behaviours? *Health Education Research*, 15(2): 131–43.

Hunt, K., Emslie, C. and Watt, G. (2000b) Barriers rooted in biography: how interpretations of family patterns of heart disease and early life experiences may undermine behavioural change in mid-life, in H. Graham (ed.) *Understanding Health Inequalities*. Buckingham: Open University Press.

Hunt, K., Ford, G., Harkins, L. and Wyke, S. (1999) Are women more ready to consult than men? Gender differences in family practitioner consultation for common chronic conditions, *Journal of Health Services Research and Policy*, 4(2): 96–100.

Jackson, D. (1990) *Unmasking Masculinity: A Critical Autobiography*. London: Unwin Hyman.

Kerssens, J.J., Bensing, J.M. and Andela, M.G. (1997) Patient preference for genders of health professionals, *Social Science and Medicine*, 44(10) 1531–40.

Kimmel, M. (1990) After fifteen years: the impact of the sociology of masculinity on the masculinity of sociology, in J. Hearn and D.H.J. Morgan (eds) *Men, Masculinities and Social Theory*. London: Unwin Hyman.

Kimmel, M. and Messner, M. (1998) *Men's Lives* (4th edn). London: Allyn & Bacon.

Kirby, R.S., Carson, C.C., Kirby, M.G. and Farah, R.N. (2004) (eds) *Men's Health* (2nd edn). London: Taylor & Francis.

Kposowa, A.J. (2000) Marital status and suicide in the National Longitudinal Mortality Study, *Journal of Epidemiology and Community Health*, 54: 254–61.

Kraemer, S. (2000) The fragile male, *British Medical Journal*, 321: 1609–12.

Lab, D.D., Feigenbaum, J.D. and De Silva P. (2000) Mental health professionals' attitudes and practices towards male childhood sexual abuse, *Child Abuse and Neglect*, 24(3): 391–409.

Lee, C. and Owens, G. (2002) *The Psychology of Men's Health*. Buckingham: Open University Press.

Lewis, C. (1986) *Becoming A Father*. Buckingham: Open University Press.

Linneman, T.J. (2000) Risk and masculinity in the everyday lives of gay men, in P. Nardi (ed.) *Gay Masculinities*. London: Sage.

Lloyd, T. (1996) *Men's Health Review*. London: Men's Health Forum.

Lloyd, T. (2001) Men and health: the context for practice, in N. Davidson and T. Lloyd (eds) *Promoting Men's Health: A Guide for Practitioners*. London: Baillière Tindall.

Lomas, L. (2003) Men at work, *Men's Health Journal*, 2(1): 4–5.

Lorber, J. and Moore, L.J. (2002) *Gender and the Social Construction of Illness* (2nd edn). Oxford: AltaMira Press.

Luck, M., Bamford, M. and Williamson, P. (2000) *Men's Health: Perspectives, Diversity and Paradox.* Oxford: Blackwell Science.

Lupton, D. (1993) Risk as moral danger: the social and political functions of risk discourse in public health, *International Journal of Health Services*, 23(3): 425–35.

Lupton, D. (1996) 'Your life in their hands': trust in the medical encounter, in J. Gabe and V. James (eds) *Health and the Sociology of Emotion.* Oxford: Blackwell.

Lupton, D. (1997) Consumerism, reflexivity and the medical encounter, *Social Science and Medicine*, 45(3): 373–81.

Lupton, D. (1998) *The Emotional Self.* London: Sage.

Lupton, D. (1999) *Risk.* London: Routledge.

Lynch, J. (1977) *Broken Heart: The Medical Consequences of Loneliness.* New York: Basic Books.

Lynch, J. (1985) *The Language of the Heart: The Human Body in Dialogue.* New York: Basic Books.

Lyng, S. (ed.) (2005) *Edgework: The Sociology of Risk-Taking.* London: Routledge.

Lyons, A.C. and Willott, S. (1999) From suet pudding to superhero: representations of men's health for women, *Health*, 3(3): 283–302.

Macintyre, S., Ford, G. and Hunt, K. (1999) Do women 'over-report' morbidity? Men's and women's responses to structured prompting on a standard question on long standing illness, *Social Science and Medicine*, 48(1): 89–98.

MacIntyre, S., Hunt, K. and Sweeting, H. (1996) Gender differences in health: are things really as simple as they seem? *Social Science and Medicine*, 42(4): 617–24.

Mair, D. (2000) The enemy within, *Counselling*, 11(7): 414–17.

Mason, O.J. and Strauss, K. (2004) Testicular cancer: passage through the help-seeking process for a cohort of UK men, *International Journal of Men's Health*, 3(2): 93–110.

McDowell, I. (1999) *Gender, Identity and Place: Understanding Feminist Geographies.* Minneapolis: University of Minnesota Press.

McDowell, L. (2002) Masculine discourses and dissonances: strutting 'lads', protest masculinity and domestic respectability, *Environment and Planning D: Society and Space*, 20: 97–119.

McGowan, F. (2002) *Idealised Fitness: the Role of the Body in Men's Biographical Narratives.* Paper given at 34th Annual Conference of the BSA Medical Sociology Group.

McVittie, C. and Willock, J. (2006) 'You can't fight windmills': how older men do health, ill-health, and masculinities, *Qualitative Health Research*, 16(6): 788–801.

Mdkeld, K. and Mustonen, H. (2000) Relationships of drinking behaviour, gender and age with reported negative and positive experiences related to drinking, *Addiction*, 95(5): 727–36.

Melluish, S. and Bulmer, D. (1999) Rebuilding solidarity: an account of a men's health action project, *Journal of Community and Applied Social Psychology*, 9: 93–100.

Men's Health Forum (2004a) *Getting it Sorted: A Policy Programme for Men's Health*. London: The Men's Health Forum.

Men's Health Forum (2004b) *2004 Briefing Paper: Men and Cancer*. London: Men's Health Forum.

Merleau-Ponty, M. (1971) *Sense and Non-sense*. Chicago: Northwestern University Press.

Miller, S. (1992) *Men and Friendship*. Los Angeles: Tarcher Inc.

Monaghan, L. (2001) Looking good feeling good: the embodied pleasure of vibrant physicality, *Sociology of Health and Illness*, 23(3): 330–56.

Morgan, D.H.J. (1981) Men, masculinity and the process of sociological enquiry, in H. Roberts (ed.) *Doing Feminist Research*. London: Routledge & Kegan Paul.

Morgan, D.H.J. (1987) 'It Will Make A Man Of You': Notes On National Service. *Masculinity and Autobiography*. Studies in Sexual Politics No.17. Manchester: University of Manchester.

Morgan, D.H.J. (1992) *Discovering Men*. London: Routledge.

Morgan, D.H.J. (1993) You too can have a body like mine: reflections on the male body and masculinities, in S. Scott and D.H.J. Morgan (eds) *Body Matters*. London: Falmer Press.

Morgan, D.H.J. and Scott, S. (1993) Bodies in a social landscape, in S. Scott and D.H.J. Morgan (eds) *Body Matters*. London: Falmer Press.

MORI (1995) *Men's Health: A Survey of District Directors of Public Health for the RCN*. London: MORI.

Moss, P. and Dyke, I. (1996) Inquiry into environment and body: women, work and chronic illness, *Environment and Planning D: Society and Space*, 14: 737–53.

Moynihan, C. (1998) Theories of masculinity, *British Medical Journal*, 317: 1072–5.

Mullen, K. (1993) *A Healthy Balance: Glaswegian Men Talking About Health, Tobacco and Alcohol*. Aldershot: Avebury.

Nardi, P. (1992) *That's What Friends are for: Friends as Family in the Gay and Lesbian Community*, in K. Plummer (ed.) *Modern Homosexualities: Fragments of Gay and Lesbian Experience*. London: Routledge.

Nettleton, S. (1995) *The Sociology of Health and Illness*. Cambridge: Polity Press.

Nettleton, S. and Bunton, R. (1995) Sociological critiques of health promotion, in R. Bunton, S. Nettleton and R. Burrows (eds) *The Sociology of Health Promotion: Critical Analysis of Consumption, Lifestyle and Risk*. London: Routledge.

Nettleton, S. and Watson, J. (1998) The body in everyday life: an introduction, in S. Nettleton and J. Watson (eds) *The Body in Everyday Life*. London: Routledge.

O'Brien, R., Hunt, K. and Hart, G. (2005) 'It's caveman stuff, but that is to a certain extent how guys still operate': men's accounts of masculinity and help seeking, *Social Science and Medicine*, 61(3): 503–16.

O'Neill, T. and Hird, M.J. (2001) Double damnation: gay disabled men and the negotiation of masculinity, in K. Backett-Milburn and L. McKie (eds) *Constructing Gendered Bodies*. Basingstoke: Palgrave.

Office for National Statistics (2002) *Living in Britain: Results from the 2001 General Household Survey*. London: The Stationery Office.

Office for National Statistics (2003) *Social Trends 33*. London: The Stationery Office.

Office for National Statistics (2005a) *Life Expectancy at Birth by Local Authority in the England and Wales 1991–1993 to 2002–2004*. London: The Stationery Office.

Office for National Statistics (2005b) *Cancer Statistics Registrations: Registrations of Cancer Diagnosed in 2002, England. Series MB1 No. 33*. London: The Stationery Office.

Office for National Statistics (2006a) Suicide trends and geographical variations in the United Kingdom 1991–2004, *Health Statistics Quarterly*, 31: 5–22.

Office for National Statistics (2006b) *Social Trends 36*. Basingstoke: Palgrave Macmillan.

Oliffe, J. and Mróz, L. (2005) Men interviewing men about health and illness: ten lessons learned, *Journal of Men's Health and Gender*, 2(2): 257–60.

Oliver, M. (1996) Defining impairment and disability: issues at stake, in C. Barns and G. Mercer (eds) *Exploring the Divide: Illness and Disability*. Leeds: The Disability Press.

Ong, B.N. and Hooper, H. (2006) Comparing clinical and lay accounts of the diagnosis and treatment of back pain, *Sociology of Health and Illness*, 28(2): 203–22.

Parish, R. (1995) Health promotion: rhetoric and reality, in R. Bunton, S. Nettleton and R. Burrows (eds) *The Sociology of Health Promotion: Critical Analysis of Consumption, Lifestyle and Risk*. London: Routledge.

Parker, I., Georgaca, E., Harper, D., McLaughlin, T. and Stowell-Smith, M. (1995) *Deconstructing Psychopathology*. London: Sage.

Parsons, T. (1964) *Essays in Sociological Theory*. London: Collier-Macmillan.

Parsons, T. and Bales, R.F. (1956) *Family, Socialization and Interaction Process*. London: Routledge & Kegan Paul.

Pateman, B. and Johnson, M. (2000) Men's lived experiences following transurethral prostatectomy for benign prostatic hypertrophy, *Journal of Advanced Nursing*, 31(1): 51–8.

Paulson, M., Danielson, E. and Söderberg, S. (2002) Struggling for a tolerable existence: the meaning of men's lived experiences of living with pain of fibromyalgia type, *Qualitative Health Research*, 12(2): 238–49.

Peate, I. (2004) Men's attitudes towards health and the implications for nursing care, *British Journal of Nursing*, 13(9): 540–5.

Peate, I. (2006) Inequality, discrimination and neglect: men's health, *British Journal of Nursing*, 15(12): 632.

Petersen, A. (1998) *Unmasking the Masculine: 'Men' and 'Identity' in a Sceptical Age*. London: Sage.

Petersen, A. and Lupton, D. (1996) *The New Public Health: Health and Self in the Age of Risk*. London: Sage.

Pill, R. and Stott, N.C.H. (1982) Concept of illness causation and responsibility: some preliminary data from a sample of working class mothers, *Social Science and Medicine*, 16: 43–52.

Piper, S. (1997) The limitations of well men clinics for health education, *Nursing Standard*, 11(30): 47–9.

Pleck, J.H. (1981) *The Myth of Masculinity*. London: MIT Press.

Pleck, J.H. (1995) The gender role strain paradigm: an update, in R.F. Levant and W.S. Pollack (eds) *A New Psychology of Men*. New York: Basic Books.

Popay, J. and Groves, K. (2000) 'Narrative' in research on gender inequalities in health, in E. Annandale and K. Hunt (eds) *Gender Inequalities in Health*. Buckingham: Open University Press.

Popay, J. and Williams, G. (1996) Public health research and lay knowledge, *Social Science and Medicine*, 42(5): 759–68.

Popay, J., Bennett, S., Thomas, C., Williams, G., Gatrell, A. and Bostock, L. (2003) Beyond 'beer, fags, egg and chips'? Exploring lay understandings of social inequalities in health, *Sociology of Health and Illness*, 25(1): 1–23.

Popay, J., Williams, G., Thomas, C. and Gatrell, T. (1998) Theorising inequalities in health: the place of lay knowledge, *Sociology of Health and Illness*, 20(5): 619–44.

Rahkonen, O., Arber, S., Lahelma, E., Martikainen, P. and Silventoinen, K. (2000) Understanding income inequalities in health among men and women in Britain and Finland, *International Journal of Health Services*, 30(1): 27–47.

Reeve, D. (2002) Negotiating the psycho-emotional dimensions of disability and their influence on identity constructions, *Disability and Society*, 17(5): 493–508.

Rhodes, T. and Cusick, L. (2000) Love and intimacy in relationship risk management: HIV positive people and their sexual partners, *Sociology of Health and Illness*, 22(1): 1–26.

Riessman, C.K. (2003) Performing identities in illness narrative: masculinity and multiple sclerosis, *Qualitative Research*, 3(1): 5–33.

Riska, E. (2002) From Type A man to the hardy man: masculinity and health, *Sociology of Health and Illness*, 24(3): 347–58.

Robertson, S. (1995) Men's health promotion in the UK: a hidden problem, *British Journal of Nursing*, 4(7): 382–401.

Robertson, S. (1998) Men's health: present practice and future hope, *British Journal of Community Nursing*, 3(1): 45–9.

Robertson, S. (2000) Middle-aged men's health, *Nursing Times*, 96(14): 43–4.

Robertson, S. (2003) 'If I let a goal in, I'll get beat up': contradictions in masculinity, sport and health, *Health Education Research*, 18(6): 706–16.

Robertson, S. (2004) Men and disability, in J. Swain, S. French, C. Barnes and C. Thomas (eds) *Disabling Barriers – Enabling Environments* (2nd edn). London: Sage.

Robertson, S. and Williams, R. (1997) *Men's Health: A Handbook for Community Health Professionals*. London: CPHVA.

Robertson, S. and Williamson, P. (2005) Men and health promotion in the UK: ten years further on? *Health Education Journal*, 64(4): 293–301.

Roos, E., Lahelma, E., Virtanen, M., Prättälä, R. and Pietinen, P. (1998) Gender, socioeconomic status and family status as determinants of food behaviour, *Social Science and Medicine*, 46(12): 1519–29.

Rosenfeld, D. and Faircloth, C.A. (2006) Medicalized masculinities: the missing link, in D. Rosenfeld, and C.A. Faircloth (eds) *Medicalized Masculinities*. Philadelphia: Temple University Press.

Roulstone, A. (2002) Disabling pasts, enabling futures? How does the changing nature of Capitalism impact on the disabled worker and jobseeker? *Disability and Society*, 17(6): 627–42.

Sabo, D. (2000) Men's health studies: origins and trends, *Journal of American College Health*, 49(3): 133–42.

Sabo, D. and Gordon, D.F. (eds) (1995) *Men's Health and Illness: Gender, Power and the Body*. London: Sage.

Saltonstall, R. (1993) Healthy bodies, social bodies: men's and women's concepts and practices of health in everyday life, *Social Science and Medicine*, 36(1): 7–14.

Sapey, B. (2000) Disablement in the informational age. *Disability and Society*, 15(4): 619–36.

Segal, L. (1997) *Slow Motion: Changing Masculinities, Changing Men* (2nd edn). London: Virago Press.

Seidler, V. (1989) *Rediscovering Masculinity: Reason, Language and Sexuality*. London: Routledge.

Seidler, V. (1992) Rejection, vulnerability, and friendship, in P. Nardi (ed.) *Men's Friendships*. London: Sage.

Seidler, V. (1994) *Unreasonable Men: Masculinity and Social Theory*. London: Routledge.

Seidler, V. (1997) *Man Enough: Embodying Masculinities*. London: Sage.

Seymour-Smith, S., Wetherell, M. and Phoenix, A. (2002) 'My wife ordered me to come': a discursive analysis of doctors' and nurses' accounts of men's use of general practitioners, *Journal of Health Psychology*, 7(3): 253–67.

Shakespeare, T. (1994). Cultural representation of disabled people: dustbins for disaowal? *Disability and Society*, 9(3): 283–99.

Shakespeare, T. (1999) When is a man not a man? When he's disabled, in J. Wild (ed.) *Working With Men for Change*. London: UCL Press.

Sharpe, S. and Arnold, S. (1999) *Men, Lifestyle and Health: A Study of Health Beliefs and Practices*. London: Social Science Research Unit, University of London.

Shilling, C. (1993) *The Body and Social Theory*. London: Sage.

Sixsmith, J. and Boneham, M. (2001) Men and masculinities: accounts of health and social capital, in C. Swann and A. Morgan (eds) *Social Capital for Health: Insights from Qualitative Research*. London: Health Development Agency.

Sixsmith, J., Boneham, M. and Goldring, J. (2001) *The Relationship Between Social Capital, Health and Gender: A Case Study of a Deprived Community.* London: Health Development Agency.

Stepney, R. (1996) Being male means being mortal, *Independent*, 8 January, p. 2.

Summer, S., Dolan, A., Thompson, V. and Hundt, G. (2002) Prostate health awareness – promoting health in the workplace, *Men's Health Journal*, 1(5): 146–8.

Thomas, C. (1999a) *Female Forms: Experiencing and Understanding Disability.* Buckingham: Open University Press.

Thomas, C. (1999b) Understanding health inequalities: the place of agency, *Health Variations Newsletter*, 3: 10–11.

Thomas, C. (2001) The body and society: some reflections on the concepts of 'disability' and 'impairment', in N. Watson and S. Cunningham-Burley (eds) *Reframing the Body*. Basingstoke: Palgrave.

Tones, K. (1997) Health education as empowerment, in M. Sidell, L. Jones, J. Katz, and A. Peberdy (eds) *Debates and Dilemmas in Promoting Health.* Buckingham: Open University Press.

Travers, K.D. (1996) The social organization of nutritional inequities, *Social Science and Medicine*, 43(4): 543–53.

Turner, B.S. (1987) *Medical Power and Social Knowledge.* London: Sage.

Turner, B.S. (1992) *Regulating Bodies: Essays in Medical Sociology.* London: Routledge.

Walker, B. and Kushner, S. (1999) The building site: an educational approach to masculine identity, *Journal of Youth Studies*, 2(1): 45–58.

Warde, A. (1992) Notes on the relationship between production and consumption, in R. Burrows and Marsh C. (eds) *Consumption and Class: Divisions and Change.* London: Macmillan.

Watson, J. (1993) Male body image and health beliefs: a qualitative study and implications for health promotion practice, *Health Education Journal*, 52(4): 246–52.

Watson, J. (2000) *Male Bodies: Health, Culture and Identity.* Buckingham: Open University Press.

Wellman, B. (1992) Men in networks: private communities, domestic friendships, in P. Nardi (ed.) *Men's Friendships.* London: Sage.

Welshman, J. (1997) 'Bringing beauty and brightness to the back streets': health education and public health in England and Wales, 1890–1940, *Health Education Journal*, 56: 199–209.

West, C. and Zimmerman, D. (1987) Doing gender, *Gender and Society*, 1(2): 125–51.

Wetherell, M. and Edley, N. (1999) Negotiating hegemonic masculinity: imaginary positions and psycho-discursive practices, *Feminism and Psychology*, 9(3): 335–56.

White, A. (1999) 'I feel a fraud': men and their experiences of acute admission following chest pain, *Nursing in Critical Care*, 4(2): 67–73.

White, A. (2001) How men respond to illness, *Men's Health Journal*, 1(1): 18–19.

White, A. (2006) Men's health in the twenty-first century, *International Journal of Men's Health*, 5(1): 1–17.

White, A. and Banks, I. (2004) Help seeking in men and the problems of late diagnosis, in R.S. Kirby, C.C. Carson, M.G. Kirby and R.N. Farah (eds) *Men's Health* (2nd edn). London: Taylor and Francis.

White, A. and Cash, K. (2003) *The State of Men's Health Across 17 European Countries*. Brussels: European Men's Health Forum.

White, A.K. and Cash, K. (2004) The state of men's health in Western Europe, *Journal of Men's Health and Gender* 1:60–6.

White, A.K. and Holmes, M. Patterns of morbidity across 44 countries among men and women aged 15–44, *Journal of Men's Health and Gender* 3(2): 139–51.

White, A. and Johnson, M. (2000) Men making sense of their chest pain: niggles, doubts and denials, *Journal of Clinical Nursing*, 9(4): 534–42.

White, C., Wiggins, R., Blane, D., Whitworth, A. and Glickman, M. (2005) Person, place or time? The effect of individual circumstances, area and changes over time on mortality in men, 1995–2001, *Health Statistics Quarterly*, 28: 18–27.

White, K. (2002) *An Introduction to the Sociology of Health and Illness*. London: Sage.

Williams, C. (2000) Doing health, doing gender: teenagers, diabetes and asthma. *Social Science and Medicine*, 50(3): 387–96.

Williams, G. (1993) Chronic illness and the pursuit of virtue in everyday life, in A. Radley (ed.) *World's of Illness: Biographical and Cultural Perspectives on Health and Disease*. London: Routledge.

Williams, R. (1983) Concepts of health: an analysis of lay logic, *Sociology*, 17: 185–204.

Williams, R. (1997) Health visitors ideologies regarding health promotion for men, *British Journal of Community Health Nursing*, 2(5): 238–48.

Williams, R. and Robertson, S. (1999) Fathers and health visitors: 'it's a secret agent thing', *Community Practitioner*, 72(3): 56–8.

Williams, R. and Robertson, S. (2006) Masculinities, men and promoting health through primary care, *Primary Health Care*, 16(8): 25–8.

Williams, S.J. (1995) Theorising class, health and lifestyles: can Bourdieu help us? *Sociology of Health and Illness*, 17(5): 577–604.

Williams, S.J. (1999) Is anybody there? Critical realism, chronic illness and the disability debate, *Sociology of Health and Illness*, 21(6): 797–819.

Williams, S.J. (2001) *Emotion in Social Theory*. London: Sage.

Williams, S.J. (2002) Corporeal reflections on the biological: reductionism, constructionism and beyond, in G. Bendelow, M. Carpenter, C. Vautier and S. Williams (eds) *Gender, Health and Healing*. London: Routledge.

Williams, S.J. (2003) Beyond meaning, discourse and the empirical world: critical realist reflections on health, *Social Theory and Health*, 1(1): 42–71.

Williams, S.J. and Bendelow, G. (1998a) *The Lived Body: Sociological Themes, Embodied Issues*. London: Routledge.

Williams, S.J. Bendelow, G. (1998b) Introduction: mapping the sociological terrain, in G. Bendelow and S.J. Williams (eds) *Emotions in Social Life: Critical Themes and Contemporary Issues*. London: Routledge.

Williams, S.J., Birke, L. and Bendelow, G. (eds) (2003) *Debating Biology: Sociological Reflections on Health, Medicine and Society*. London: Routledge.

Williamson, P. (1995) Their own worst enemy, *Nursing Times*, 91(48): 25–7.

World Health Organization (2001) *Mainstreaming Gender Equity in Health: The Need to Move Forward*. Copenhagen: WHO Regional Office for Europe.

Yamey, G. (2000) Health minister announces initiatives on men's health, *British Medical Journal*, 320: 961.

Zaninotto, P., Wardle, H., Stamatakis, E., Mindell, J. and Head, J. (2006) *Forecasting Obesity to 2010*. London: Department of Epidemiology and Public Health, Royal Free and University College Medical School.

Index